Y0-BQI-783

Gaining Cultural Competence in Career Counseling

Gaining Cultural Competence in Career Counseling

KATHY EVANS

University of South Carolina

Lahaska Press
Houghton Mifflin Company
Boston ■ *New York*

This book is dedicated to my parents, Dr. Ruppert L. Evans and Mrs. Marie Evans, who have been unwaveringly supportive of my endeavors throughout my life.

Publisher, Lahaska Press: Barry Fetterolf
Senior Editor, Lahaska Press: Mary Falcon
Senior Marketing Manager, Lahaska Press: Barbara LeBuhn
Associate Project Editor: Deborah Berkman
Art and Design Manager: Gary Crespo
Cover Design Manager: Anne S. Katzeff
Composition Buyer: Chuck Dutton
New Title Project Manager: Susan Brooks-Peltier
Editorial Assistant: Evangeline Bermas

Cover image: © Blinkstock

For instructors who want more information about Lahaska Press books and teaching aids, contact the Houghton Mifflin Faculty Services Center at
    Tel: 800-733-1717, x4034
    Fax: 800-733-1810

Or visit us on the Web at **www.lahaskapress.com**.

Credits

Figure 1.1 Reprinted from Arredonde, Patricia; Toporek, Rebecca; Brown, Sherlon Pack; Jones, Janet; Lock, Don C.; Sanchez, Joe; Stadler, Holly. (1996). Operationalization of the Multicultural Counseling Competencies. *Journal of Counseling and Development,* 24, 57–73. Copyright © 1996 The American Counseling Association. Reprinted with permission. No further reproduction authorized without written permission from the American Counseling Association.

Figure 1.2 Reproduced with permission from NCDA.

Figure 2.1 From "Eliminating Cultural Oppression in Counseling: Toward a General Theory," by D. W. Sue, 1978, *Journal of Counseling Psychology,* Vol. 25, p. 422. Copyright © 1978 American Psychological Association. Adapted with permission.

Credits appear on page 199, which constitute a continuation of the copyright page.

Copyright © 2008 by Houghton Mifflin Company. All rights reserved.

Lahaska Press, established as an imprint of Houghton Mifflin Company in 1999, is dedicated to publishing textbooks and instructional media for counseling and the helping professions. Its editorial offices are located in the small town of Lahaska, Pennsylvania. *Lahaska* is a Native American Lenape word meaning "source of much writing."

No part of this work may be reproduced or transmitted in any form or by any means, electronic or mechanical, including photocopying and recording, or by any information storage or retrieval system without the prior written permission of Houghton Mifflin Company unless such copying is expressly permitted by federal copyright law. Address inquiries to College Permissions, Houghton Mifflin Company, 222 Berkeley Street, Boston, MA 02116-3764.

Printed in the U.S.A.

Library of Congress Control Number: 2006938434

ISBN-10: 0-618-57358-5
ISBN-13: 978-0-618-57358-5

123456789-VHO-11 10 09 08 07

Contents

CHAPTER 8   Social Action   171

PREFACE

For career counseling professionals to be considered proficient in the field, they must master two sets of competencies: the Career Counseling Competencies developed by The National Career Development Association (NCDA) and the multicultural counseling competencies developed by the Association for Multicultural Counseling and Development (AMCD). Unfortunately, these two areas of competence are taught separately in training, and professionals are given little guidance as to how to integrate them.

The lack of synthesis of the competencies becomes especially worrisome when students' practicum and internship experiences do not include diverse clients and/or multiculturally trained supervisors. In a worst case scenario, when synthesis of competencies does not occur, career counselors will enter the field and approach their culturally diverse clients from an ethnocentric, monocultural, one-size-fits all perspective (Sue, et al., 1998).

Gaining Cultural Competence in Career Counseling is designed to help counselors and counselors-in-training acquire competence simultaneously in both career counseling and multicultural counseling. The goal of this book is not only to describe the philosophical reasons for practicing culturally appropriate career counseling, but also to provide counselors with concrete ideas on how to implement those philosophies. To accomplish this task, I have integrated the original AMCD competencies (Arredondo, et al., 1996), the most recent AMCD update (Roysircar, et al., 2003), and the APA multicultural guidelines (APA, 2003), and have broadened the definition of the term *multicultural* to include not only racial and ethnic minority groups, but also other oppressed groups (such as white women, persons with disabilities, and Gay, Lesbian, Bisexual, and Transgendered (GLBT). Finally, I have included a chapter on social action, to recognize and encourage this growing movement among multicultural counselors.

CONTENT AND ORGANIZATION

In essence, the book is divided into two parts. The first part is comprised of four chapters that focus on the foundational skills for effective counseling across cultures. The second part integrates those multicultural competencies with specific career counseling competencies. It is crucial for counselors and counselors-in-training to master the multicultural skills presented in the first part of the book before moving ahead to the applications addressed in the second part. Following is a more specific guide to each chapter.

Chapter 1, The Importance of Culturally Competent Career Counseling

The first chapter sets the tone for the rest of the book, beginning with a provocative scenario that helps students understand the expanded definition of multiculturalism employed in this book. The chapter highlights the various reasons why multicultural counseling is important, introduces the AMCD multicultural counseling competencies (included in abbreviated form as Figure 1.1) and NCDA Career Counseling Competencies (included in their entirety as Figure 1.2), discusses via illustrated examples how the ethical codes of the ACA, APA, and NCDA speak to the importance of multiculturalism, and begins the process of synthesizing the AMCD and NCDA competencies.

Chapter 2, Awareness of Your Own Cultural Heritage

This chapter leads readers through an exploration of their own cultural heritages, through a discussion of the dominant American culture, and definitions of cultural relativism, worldview, and value orientation. Readers are introduced to the Racial/Cultural Identity Development Model and the White Racial Identity Model. The chapter provides a wide variety of exercises to facilitate independent self-exploration of cultural heritage.

Chapter 3, Your Biases

For some readers, this may be the book's most emotionally challenging chapter, for it encourages counselors and counselors-in-training to uncover their own biases and to consider how these biases manifest themselves in stereotyping, prejudice, racism and oppression, and privilege. As in Chapter 2, plentiful exercises facilitate reader self-exploration. Once biases are identified, counselors are encouraged to determine ways in which their biases may impact their work with clients who differ from them.

Chapter 4, Awareness of the Client's Worldviews

The final foundational chapter in the book, Chapter 4 asks readers who have just explored their own cultures and own biases to step out of themselves and focus on the worldviews of clients, worldviews that can be better understood when counselors and counselors-in-training understand the client's history, the client's degree of cultural mistrust, the client's cultural expectations and values, the client's difference from others within his or her cultural group, and the client's racial/cultural identity development status. The chapter then relates these various factors to the career counseling experience and concludes with on overview of current sociopolitical issues that affect client worldviews and attitudes toward work today, such as affirmative action, the current state of GLBT and women's rights, the Americans with Disabilities Act, and the current situation with regard to poverty and welfare.

Chapter 5, Using Career Development Theories

As the first step in the application of the multicultural skills explored in the first half of the book, the second half commences with a discussion of the effectiveness and ineffectiveness of various career development theories, in terms of multicultural application. This chapter analyzes the traditional career theories, including Parson's trait and factor theory, Super's career development theory, Holland's career theory of personality types and environments, and Krumboltz's social learning theory of career development. Current theories that more strongly represent diversity, such as Gottfredson's developmental model for counseling and Social Cognitive Career Theory, are also discussed, along with recent career counseling process models specifically designed for multicultural groups.

Chapter 6, Cultural Competence in Testing

This chapter discusses the strengths and limitations of existing career tests—including interest inventories, aptitude tests, and personality tests—and provides suggestions for the appropriate selection, administration, and interpretation of standardized tests with multicultural populations. In addition, the chapter explores various cultural and environmental factors that may affect test outcomes, such as values and beliefs, race/ethnicity/sexual orientation/gender, cultural/racial identity, acculturation and language, socioeconomic status, community, and racism and discrimination. As a means of concretizing the discussion, a single case study is followed throughout the chapter.

Chapter 7, Multiculturally Competent Career Counseling Skills

Beginning with a review of the NCDA and AMCD competencies, this chapter integrates the career and multicultural competencies in a clear and straightforward manner. The integration is followed by a close examination of the synthesis of career and multicultural competencies in practice. Each of the eight stages of career counseling is examined in detail, with an ongoing case study woven throughout the discussion to illustrate real-world applications.

Chapter 8, Social Action

Understanding and applying multiculturalism in a career counseling context has been the focus of the book up to this point. This chapter takes multicultural career counseling to the next logical step, one that isn't often discussed in career textbooks. It advocates moving from *reacting* to the occupational oppression of multicultural individuals to *acting*, that is, making positive changes to the social systems in order to reduce occupational oppression in the future. The chapter introduces the importance of social action and discusses in detail the eight social action skills categories for career counselors to master, as designed by C. C. Lee and G. R. Walz.

SPECIAL FEATURES

I have included a number of special features in this book to supplement the discussion and promote active learning, the end result of which I hope will be enhanced actual career counselor practice with culturally diverse clients The special features are as follows:

- *Exercises:* Most chapters, particularly those in the first portion of the book where the focus is on the development of multicultural skills, include extensive exercises to help readers internalize the chapter content.
- *Real-World Examples and Scenarios:* All of the chapters include real-world examples and scenarios to bring to life the abstract concepts being discussed.
- *"Final Thoughts"* and *"Review/Reflection Questions":* The Final Thoughts and end-of-chapter Review/Reflection Questions have been included to reinforce key chapter material before moving on to the next chapter.
- *References:* Each chapter concludes with a list of works cited within the chapter, enabling readers to further explore various topics if they so wish.

ACKNOWLEDGEMENTS

My sincere and heart-felt gratitude goes to my good friends Marva Larrabee, Ann Addison, Caroline Hair, Deanna Moore, and Sherman Lane, who helped me write this book by listening to me, brainstorming with me, and helping me to keep my life on track in more ways than I can mention.

My graduate assistants Alexanderia Smith and Matthew Lemberger helped me keep my classes going, while I wrote, by keeping track of assignments, and they helped me keep my writing on schedule by spending many hours searching the literature, returning overdue books, and proofreading everything.

I am thankful for the support of my Department Chairs, Jim Carper and Alan Wieder, for allowing me to have extra time with graduate assistants during this project, and I am thankful for my fellow faculty, who were supportive, cooperative, and flexible enough to juggle responsibilities with me during this time.

I am especially indebted to my long-time friends and colleagues Beth Kincade and Susan Seem for tolerating my putting our joint writing commitments in slow motion while I worked on this project.

I am extremely grateful to my fellow counselors, my students, their site supervisors, and their clients, whose stories inspired the scenarios and real examples. Many, many thanks to the following manuscript reviewers who carefully assessed drafts of this book and provided detailed and thoughtful comments to help keep the book on track and in focus:

Lakota L. Brown, Northern Arizona University
Alan Burkard, Marquette University

LuAnnette T. Butler, Austin Peay State University
Y. Barry Chung, University of Georgia
Jelane A. Kennedy, College of St. Rose
Lee Covington Rush, North Dakota State University
Anthony T. Strange, University of Alaska, Fairbanks

Mary Falcon, Senior Editor of Lahaska Press, was the impetus for this project, and her incredible patience, encouragement, and faith in me is why this text even exists. I also want to thank Bruce Cantley, Developmental Editor, for his hard work in smoothing out the rough edges of the manuscript and helping it reach its final form.

K.E.

CHAPTER 1
The Importance of Culturally Competent Career Counseling

Mary Speaks, a twenty-five-year-old, single, European American woman has been a career counselor for five months at a nonprofit organization in the southeastern region of the United States that offers a variety of counseling services to the community. Mary is proud of her multicultural competence in working with people of color, who make up 40 percent of her client load. Recently, she received a folder for a new client—a thirty-eight-year-old European American married man, Joe, who was out of work due to a factory closing. He had two children and a wife who worked at a retail chain store. Mary was surprised to see that at his age, Joe still had not completed high school. The agency provides a three-year federal grant to assist low-income, displaced workers to retrain and reenter the workforce. This man was Mary's first white client eligible for assistance through this grant.

When Mary first met Joe, it appeared to her as if he hadn't bathed in some time. The T-shirt he was wearing barely covered his ample abdomen and, to her horror, a confederate flag was emblazoned on the front. Mary could not take her eyes off the T-shirt during the first ten minutes of the session. The client spoke loudly and often interrupted her when she spoke. He called her honey in almost every sentence, and often challenged the information she gave him. When Mary informed Joe that the agency required that all participants enroll in a GED program, the client replied, "Well, honey, you just let them know that I ain't gonna do that. I'll be damned if I'm gonna sit in some classroom with a bunch of niggers and spics like you got in that waiting room. I just wanna get into one of them apprenticeship programs—what they told me you have here, and I don't wanna waste no time doing that *#! GED." This statement made Mary so angry that she could barely stand to *stay in the same room with this man. She thought he was rude, arrogant, and a racist pig—a real redneck. However, she just bit the inside of her mouth and continued with the interview. Her questions and probes became fewer and fewer until it was time for the session to end.*

Mary had never disliked a client so much, and she was surprised at her raw emotions with him. She didn't see how she could continue working with him and told her peer supervisor that she was tempted to "haul off and smack" him. Mary thought it was in the best interest of the client to refer him to another counselor. She personally didn't see how the agency could take on such a client.

In the above scenario, Mary has met a new challenge to her multicultural sensitivity as a counselor. Mary had previously assumed that multiculturalism only involved being sensitive to and accepting of people who were racially different from her. Even though Mary and her client were of the same racial heritage, there were cultural and class differences that were significant enough to ignite anger in her. Mary fell victim to what Pedersen (1984) identified as one of the ten most "frequently encountered examples of cultural biases" in counseling (p. 46)—presuming that she was fully aware of all of her cultural assumptions. As Mary learned when she encountered someone who, though of the same race, was from a completely different world in terms of class and culture, counselors need to be continuously vigilant of their biases and prejudices in order to be sensitive to clients from all types of backgrounds. Mary's client, though obviously and reprehensively racist and sexist, was also undereducated and poor—aspects of the client that were overshadowed in Mary's mind by his prejudices and that prevented her from considering his qualifications to receive the agency's services. To avoid overlooking areas of bias such as those described above, most practitioners, educators, and researchers embrace a more inclusive definition of multicultural counseling (Arredondo et al., 1996; Das, 1995; Sue et al., 1998). In this text, I, too, adopt a broad definition of multicultural counseling that includes not only race, culture, and ethnicity, but also gender, sexual orientation, physical ability status, age, and class. My definition of multicultural counseling is not so broad as to say that all counseling is multicultural. Nevertheless, in a counseling relationship, the potential for differences between the persons involved—whether they be racial, ethnic, gender, sexual orientation, class, age and/or ability in nature—are considerable and require that counselors undergo special training to be effective.

You are reading this book to strengthen your career counseling skills in a variety of ways with people who are different from you. It is my wish that by reading this book, you will become more competent and more confident in handling issues of multiculturalism and diversity. This chapter will introduce you to the reasons why multicultural counseling is a necessary subject, then generally describe both the multicultural and career counseling competencies that will be examined more closely in subsequent chapters, and finally discuss the importance of ethics within the multicultural career counseling setting.

WHY MULTICULTURAL COUNSELING?

For years now, the counseling and psychology literature has forecast the impact of the growth in ethnic minority populations in the U.S. on the helping professions. As of this writing, we have come face to face with the reality of the diversity of this country. The United States is populated by so many different groups of people today that it has become difficult for the government to classify and count them all. The Census Bureau has gone from listing only two categories for race in 1960 to listing fourteen categories in 2000, with the option of identifying with more than one group (www.census.gov). In the 2000 census, 24.9 percent of the respondents indicated that they were of a race other than "white only." More than 30 percent of the population of eight states was non-white, and in six of the ten largest U.S. cities, more than half of the population was non-white (www.census.gov). Although racial differences tell only part of the story where multicultural counseling competence is concerned, these numbers give us some insight into the enormity of the issue of multiculturalism.

The following vignette, from a European American female community college career counselor, further illustrates the importance of multicultural career counseling in a real-world context:

I remember the first time I realized the importance of my multicultural training. It was a day in early August, and things were really picking up in our office just before the start of the semester. My first client was a young European American mother of three whose husband had been laid off from a construction job. The couple did not know when or if he would find employment again. She needed to find a higher-paying job than her minimum wage position at a restaurant. When she left, I saw a disabled African American male college graduate who was also looking to find a new career that would make better use of his talents than his work as a shoe salesman. He thought he could make a lot more money in a technical career. I also saw an Asian American female high school senior who was distraught because she wanted to attend the community college for specific career training but her parents were adamant that she attend a prestigious four-year college nearby. My last client of the day was a thirty-year-old lesbian Latina. Her current career was as a fourth grade teacher, but she was afraid she would lose her job when she came out of the closet. She didn't feel up to a fight with the school board so she wanted to prepare for an alternative career.

I never thought that I would see so many people who differed from me so significantly. Certainly I never fathomed that it would happen in one day. I was thankful that day that I was able to meet most of the needs of my clients, but the experience reminded me that I would need to continue to educate myself about cultural and other differences, and that I would need to continue to explore my own biases and prejudices.

Research shows that ethnic minority clients appreciate and respond well to multicultural content in counseling. Such content helps to build counselor credibility and is linked to the client's willingness to continue in counseling (Burkard, Knox, Groen, Perez & Hess, 2006; Maxie, Arnold & Stephenson, 2006; Thompson & Jenal, 1994). Conversely, counseling that avoids multicultural issues has proven to be detrimental. In their research, Thompson and Jenal found that ethnic minority clients of counselors who avoided the topic of race during counseling tended to become disengaged during the counseling process. To increase multicultural counseling competence and to meet the needs of ethnic minority groups, counselor preparation programs have been offering training in multicultural counseling for more than twenty years. The number of programs offering training has increased dramatically in recent years due, in part, to the insistence of multicultural advocates

(Sue et al., 1998). Today, programs accredited by the American Psychological Association (APA) and the Council for the Accreditation of Counseling and Related Educational Programs (CACREP) must include coursework on sociocultural foundations (APA, 2002a; CACREP, 2001).

Researchers in multicultural counseling have criticized training that consists of a single course rather than an infusion of multicultural content throughout the curriculum (Falicov, 1995; Ridley et al., 1997; Tomlinson-Cole & Wang, 1999). Programs that offer a single multicultural counseling course may be running under the assumption that students should be able to apply their multicultural counseling knowledge to all of the other courses in the curriculum. However, little evidence has been brought forth that this kind of overlap in knowledge actually occurs. Critics of the one-course strategy believe that if the course depends heavily on written material rather than experiential learning, students will be unable to acquire deeper levels of understanding of cultural differences. For instance, Sue and colleagues (1992) and others have suggested that when students receive a purely intellectual treatment of multicultural counseling, they fail to appreciate the sociopolitical context of their clients' lives. They need to have more than an intellectual understanding of oppression, discrimination, and racism (Ridley et al., 1997). To be multiculturally competent, the trainees must internalize this information. They need to read about it, experience it, and hear about it in every class as well as apply the skills in practicum and internship settings. A recent national survey of counselor training programs reported that 89 percent of the counseling doctoral programs studied offer at least one multicultural counseling course, 58 percent stated that they integrate multicultural issues in all their courses, and 35 percent state that students work with a multicultural clientele in practicum and internship experiences (Ponterotto, 1997). These figures tell us that there is still a long way to go before all counselors are trained to be truly multiculturally competent.

The results of the Ponterotto (1997) survey suggest that a large number of trainees have not had multicultural training that was infused into their entire curriculum. It is reasonable to assume, therefore, that there are a number of career development professionals who have not been trained to combine their skills in career development with those in multicultural counseling. Many currently available texts used by instructors in graduate training programs often devote only a single chapter to multicultural issues or special populations (Evans & Larrabee, 2002). Similarly, multicultural texts rarely contain information related to career development (Evans & Rotter, 2000). In 1993, the issue of raising the multicultural career counseling competence level of counselor trainees was addressed in a special edition of the *Career Development Quarterly.* While much has been written about career counseling of diverse populations in the decade since that publication, there is little evidence of specific training in multicultural career counseling.

To be multiculturally effective with all clients, career counselors must be able to synthesize multicultural and career competencies. Given that multicultural counseling and career counseling are taught separately, there are few opportunities for synthesis. This failure to synthesize knowledge and skills is especially worrisome when students' practicum and internship experiences do not include a diverse clientele and a multiculturally trained supervisor. The worse case scenario is when synthesis does not occur, a counselor will approach his or her culturally different clients from an ethnocentric, monocultural, one-size-fits all perspective. Such a counselor would not vary career counseling processes or techniques with clients regardless of their race, ethnicity, religion, age, or sexual orientation; and the client may suffer as a consequence (Sue et al., 1998). The goal of this text is to help counselors discover ways to bring together their skills in career counseling with those of multicultural counseling. I believe a blending of the multicultural and career counseling competencies will accomplish this goal.

MULTICULTURAL COMPETENCIES

The first attempt to formalize multicultural competencies was made by the APA Division of Counseling Psychology Committee on Cross-Cultural Competencies (Sue et al., 1982). The committee, led by Derald Wing Sue, published the first list of eleven multicultural counseling competencies. These competencies have become the foundation of subsequent competency statements that have been continually approved by counseling organizations (Ponterotto, Fuertes & Chin, 2000; Sue et al., 1998). Derald Sue also headed the competency writing committee of the Association for Multicultural Counseling and Development (AMCD), a division of the American Counseling Association (ACA). He was given the charge to further develop the original eleven competencies. This refinement of the competencies was published in 1992 and included thirty-one different competencies (Sue et al., 1992). Six divisions of ACA, Association for Counselor Education and Supervision (ACES); the Association for Adult Development and Aging (ADA); the American School Counselor Association (ASCA); the Association for Gay, Lesbian, and Bisexual Issues in Counseling (AGLBIC); the Association for Specialists in Group Work (ASGW); the International Association of Marriage and Family Counseling (IAMFC); and two divisions of APA (Division 17 and 45) have endorsed these competencies. The AMCD and APA's Division of Counseling Psychology have continued to update and perfect the competency statements. When the competencies were criticized for being too vague to be included in the accreditation standards, Arredondo et al. (1996) tackled the enormous task of operationalizing them. In the resulting document, each competency was broken down into several explanatory statements that described the specific behaviors counselors need to master in order to achieve multicultural competence. The authors also included strategies for achieving these competencies. The competencies were updated in 2003, and the work in the previous document has been extended to include case studies and practical examples, organizational plans, and with more resent research findings (Roysircar et al., 2003).

In 1998, Sue and a joint committee of the Division of Counseling Psychology and the Society for the Psychological Study of Ethnic Minority Issues further expanded the competencies to include multicultural organizational competence. The most recent effort to update the competencies was published by the American Psychological Association in 2002, entitled "Guidelines on Multicultural Education, training, research, practice, and organizational change for Psychologists" (www.apa.org/pi/multiculturalguidelines/homepage.html). The update differs from the association's previous (1990) document in that "it is the first to address the implications of race and ethnicity in psychological education training, research, practice, and organizational change" (p. 14). The guidelines are scheduled to expire in 2009 in order that new research, legislation, and practices that emerge may be included at that time.

In this book, emphasis will be placed on the Arredondo and colleagues (1996) publication, whose competency statements are outlined in Figure 1.1. The entire document, competencies, and explanatory statements may be found in the original journal article. While the new APA *Guidelines* have included more recent developments in the organizational arena, the authors note that they have narrowly defined the term "multicultural" to "refer to interactions between individuals from minority ethnic and racial groups in the U.S. and the dominant European-American culture" (p. 2). The broad nature of the AMCD competencies is consistent with the goals of this text in that they address the multiple ways that individuals define themselves, beyond race and ethnicity.

Arredondo and colleagues (1996) outline three dimensions of personal identity, which take into account not only racial and cultural differences in people but also other differences that are important in peoples' lives. The outline assigns a separate letter designation to each of the three dimensions. Dimension A includes "characteristics that serve as profile for all people" (p. **47**)—and includes those characteristics that are predetermined in people—age, gender, culture, ethnicity, race, and language. The B dimension includes those aspects of a person's identity that may be influenced by the A dimension or by history and experience. They include: educational background, geographic location, relationship status, religion, work experience, and hobbies and recreation. The C dimension encompasses those characteristics that are universal but that may affect individuals differently, such as historical, political, and sociocultural events. "The model communicates several premises: (a) that we are all multicultural individuals; (b) that we all possess a personal, political, and historical culture; (c) that we are affected by sociocultural political environment and historical events; and (d) that multiculturalism also interacts with multiple factors of individual diversity" (p. 3). Arredondo and colleagues (1996) suggest that all three dimensions must be addressed in counseling and that to address two of the dimensions and not the third would undermine the counseling relationship. Counselors who tend to ignore the C dimension, for example, even though they can communicate their acceptance of cultural differences may miss important client issues. A Christian counselor who is seeing an Arab Muslim may be accepting of the differences between the client and himself or herself. But if the counselor does not address the effects on the client of negative U.S. sentiments towards Arabs and Muslims during counseling, the client may think the topic is forbidden, thereby creating a barrier in the relationship.

The issues receiving the most attention in multicultural counseling literature in recent years have been in organizational multicultural competence and in social justice. Partly, the increased interest in organizational multicultural competence may be due to the increasing number of ethnic minority clients utilizing community mental health centers, and to the difficulties encountered by these clients within this setting. As mental health counselors gained more training in cultural sensitivity, they

---

Figure 1.1   AMCD Cross-Cultural Competencies and Objectives

I. Counselor Awareness of Own Cultural Values and Biases
   A.   Attitudes and Beliefs
      1. Culturally skilled counselors believe that cultural self-awareness and sensitivity to one's own cultural heritage is essential.
      2. Culturally skilled counselors are aware of how their own cultural background and experiences have influenced attitudes, values, and biases about psychological processes.
      3. Culturally skilled counselors are able to recognize the limits of their multicultural competency and expertise.
      4. Culturally skilled counselors recognize their sources of discomfort with differences that exist between themselves and clients in terms of race, ethnicity and culture.

   B.   Knowledge
      1. Culturally skilled counselors have specific knowledge about their own racial and cultural heritage and how it personally and professionally affects their definitions of and biases about normality/abnormality and the process of counseling.
      2. Culturally skilled counselors possess knowledge and understanding about how oppression, racism, discrimination, and stereotyping affect them personally and in their work. This allows individuals to acknowledge their own racist attitudes, beliefs, and feelings. Although this standard applies to all groups, for White counselors it may mean that they understand how they may have directly or indirectly benefited from individual, institutional, and cultural racism as outlined in White identity development models.
      3. Culturally skilled counselors possess knowledge about their social impact on others. They are knowledgeable about communication style differences, how their style may clash with or foster the counseling process with persons of color or others different from themselves based on the A, B, and C, Dimensions, and how to anticipate the impact it may have on others.

   C.   Skills
      1. Culturally skilled counselors seek out educational, consultative, and training experiences to improve their understanding and effectiveness in working with culturally different populations. Being able to recognize the limits of their competencies, they (a) seek consultation, (b) seek further training or education, (c) refer out to more qualified individuals or resources, or (d) engage in a combination of these.
      2. Culturally skilled counselors are constantly seeking to understand themselves as racial and cultural beings and are actively seeking a nonracist identity.

II. Counselor Awareness of Client's Worldview
   A.   Attitudes and Beliefs
      1. Culturally skilled counselors are aware of their negative and positive emotional reactions toward other racial and ethnic groups that may prove detrimental to the counseling relationship. They are willing to contrast their own beliefs and attitudes with those of their culturally different clients in a nonjudgmental fashion.
      2. Culturally skilled counselors are aware of their stereotypes and preconceived notions that they may hold toward other racial and ethnic minority groups.

   B.   Knowledge
      1. Culturally skilled counselors possess specific knowledge and information about the particular group with which they are working. They are aware of the life experiences, cultural heritage, and

continued

Figure 1.1   *continued*

historical background of their culturally different clients. This particular competency is strongly linked to the "minority identity development models" available in the literature.

2. Culturally skilled counselors understand how race, culture, ethnicity, and so forth may affect personality formation, vocational choices, manifestation of psychological disorders, help-seeking behavior, and the appropriateness or inappropriateness of counseling approaches.

3. Culturally skilled counselors understand and have knowledge about sociopolitical influences that impinge upon the life of racial and ethnic minorities. Immigration issues, poverty, racism, stereotyping, and powerlessness may impact self esteem and self concept in the counseling process.

C. Skills

1. Culturally skilled counselors should familiarize themselves with relevant research and the latest findings regarding mental health and mental disorders of various ethnic and racial groups. They should actively seek out educational experiences that enrich their knowledge, understanding, and cross-cultural skills for more effective counseling behavior.

2. Culturally skilled counselors become actively involved with minority individuals outside the counseling setting (e.g., community events, social and political functions, celebrations, friendships, neighborhood groups, and so forth) so that their perspective of minorities is more than an academic or helping exercise.

III. Culturally Appropriate Intervention Strategies

A. Beliefs and Attitudes

1. Culturally skilled counselors respect clients' religious and/or spiritual beliefs and values, including attributions and taboos, because they affect worldview, psychosocial functioning, and expressions of distress.

2. Culturally skilled counselors respect indigenous helping practices and respect help-giving networks among communities of color.

3. Culturally skilled counselors value bilingualism and do not view another language as an impediment to counseling (monolingualism may be the culprit).

B. Knowledge

1. Culturally skilled counselors have a clear and explicit knowledge and understanding of the generic characteristics of counseling and therapy (culture bound, class bound, and monolingual) and how they may clash with the cultural values of various cultural groups.

2. Culturally skilled counselors are aware of institutional barriers that prevent minorities from using mental health services.

3. Culturally skilled counselors have knowledge of the potential bias in assessment instruments and use procedures and interpret findings in a way that recognize the cultural and linguistic characteristics of the clients.

4. Culturally skilled counselors have knowledge of minority family structures, hierarchies, values, and beliefs from various cultural perspectives. They are knowledgeable about the community where a particular cultural group may reside and the resources in the community.

5. Culturally skilled counselors should be aware of relevant discriminatory practices at the social and community level that may be affecting the psychological welfare of the population being served.

C. Skills

1. Culturally skilled counselors are able to engage in a variety of verbal and nonverbal helping responses. They are able to send and receive both verbal and non-verbal messages accurately and

---

Figure 1.1 *continued*

---

appropriately. They are not tied down to only one method or approach to helping, but recognize that helping styles and approaches may be culture bound. When they sense that their helping style is limited and potentially inappropriate, they can anticipate and modify it.

2. Culturally skilled counselors are able to exercise institutional intervention skills on behalf of their clients. They can help clients determine whether a "problem" stems from racism or bias in others (the concept of health paranoia) so that clients do not inappropriately personalize problems.

3. Culturally skilled counselors are not averse to seeking consultation with traditional healers or religious and spiritual leaders and practitioners in the treatment of culturally different clients when appropriate.

4. Culturally skilled counselors take responsibility for interacting in the language requested by the client and, if not feasible, make appropriate referrals. A serious problem arises when the linguistic skills of a counselor do not match the language of the client. This being the case, counselors should (a) seek a translator with cultural knowledge and appropriate professional background or (b) refer to a knowledgeable and competent bilingual counselor.

5. Culturally skilled counselors have training and expertise in the use of traditional assessment and testing instruments. They not only understand the technical aspects of the instruments but are also aware of the cultural limitations. This allows them to use test instruments for the welfare of different clients.

6. Culturally skilled counselors should attend to as well as work to eliminate biases, prejudices, and discriminatory contexts in conducting evaluations and providing interventions and should develop sensitivity to issues of oppression, sexism, heterosexism, elitism, and racism.

7. Culturally skilled counselors take responsibility for educating their clients to the processes of psychological intervention, such as goals, expectations, legal rights, and the counselor's orientation.

From: Arredondo, et al., 1996 pp. 57–73

---

found that they were often fighting against a system that was designed for a much different, mostly white, population. It became clear that mental health organizations themselves, not just the individuals working in these organizations, needed to become more multiculturally competent. Similarly, employers in business and industry have faced the reality of an increasingly multicultural workforce and with the requirements of Equal Pay Act of 1963 (which gives protection against gender bias in wages) and affirmative action (which requires employers to be proactive in hiring and promoting ethnic minorities, white women, and people with disabilities). Employers have spearheaded many of the efforts to help their organizations become more multiculturally competent.

The increased focus on social justice may be a result of the work of Vera and Speight (2003), who criticized the multicultural counseling competencies for failing to attend to issues of social justice, and they called for the inclusion of skills required to act as institutional, agency, and societal change agents. According to Arredondo and Perez (2003), "social justice has always been the core of the multicultural competency movement" (p. 282). The social justice and multicultural counseling competence are intertwined and interdependent.

CAREER COUNSELING COMPETENCIES

Because this book is not just about multicultural competency but more specifically about multicultural competency in a career counseling setting, it is vital to understand the career counseling competencies in conjunction with multicultural competencies. The career counseling competencies referred to in this book are those that were created, refined, and disseminated by the National Career Development Association (NCDA). Under their previous name, the National Vocational Guidance Association (NVGA), this organization completed the first set of career counseling competencies in 1981 (NVGA, 1982). The goal was to define the counselor's role in career counseling. This document described six competency areas—general counseling, information, individual and group assessment, management and administration, implementation, and consultation. The original publication of these competencies was aimed specifically at professional counselors at or above the master's level, and they made a significant statement regarding the minimum skills professional counselors needed to acquire if they wished to engage in career counseling. Over time, the competencies became the basis for accreditation and certification of career counselors (Engels et al., 1995). The NCDA has continued to update and review the career counseling competencies. In 1991, they updated the competency areas and broadened them. Not only were five new categories added but also the existing categories were refined to include minimum skills. The five new categories were career development theory, special populations, supervision, ethical and legal issues, and research evaluation (Herr, Cramer & Niles, 2004). The most recent revision of the competency areas was published in 1997 (NCDA, 1997). In this revision, the competency statements were further refined. Some categories were renamed, and technology was added as a new category. Under each of the competencies, statements identifying the specific skills and the knowledge base needed to meet the competency requirement were added. The NCDA intended that the competencies would be used for training new counselors and for practicing counselors to use if they wanted to add career counseling as an area of expertise (NCDA, 1997). The most recent NCDA competencies are outlined in Figure 1.2. A complete breakdown of the competencies may be found in Appendix B.

Many counselor preparation programs require students to take courses that teach most of the competencies listed above. For example, counseling programs typically require courses in research, assessment, individual and group counseling, and diverse populations, and many programs offer courses in ethics, consultation, and supervision. However, just as in multicultural counseling, students need practicum or internship experience to truly develop the skills needed for competency in career counseling. The ideal situation would be for trainees to get practical career counseling experience with diverse groups of people. The expertise counselors gain by becoming culturally competent in career counseling will increase the likelihood that they will act ethically with their culturally different clients.

Figure 1.2 National Career Development Association (NCDA) Career Counseling Competencies and Performance Indicators, Revised Version, 1997

Career Development Theory	Theory base and knowledge considered essential for professionals engaging in career counseling and development. Demonstration of knowledge of

1. Counseling theories and associated techniques
2. Theories and models of career development
3. Individual differences related to gender, sexual orientation, race, ethnicity, and physical and mental capacities
4. Theoretical models for career development and associated counseling and information-delivery techniques and resources
5. Human growth and development throughout the life span
6. Role relationships that facilitate life-work planning
7. Information, techniques, and models related to career planning and placement

Individual and Group Counseling Skills	Individual and group counseling competencies considered essential to effective career counseling. Demonstration of ability to

1. Establish and maintain productive personal relationships with individuals
2. Establish and maintain a productive group climate
3. Collaborate with clients in identifying personal goals
4. Identify and select techniques appropriate to client or group goals and client needs, psychological states, and developmental tasks
5. Identify and understand clients' personal characteristics related to career
6. Identify and understand social contextual conditions affecting clients' careers
7. Identify and understand familial, subcultural and cultural structures and functions as they are related to clients' careers
8. Identify and understand clients' career decision-making processes
9. Identify and understand clients' attitudes toward work and workers
10. Identify and understand clients' biases toward work and workers based on gender, race, and cultural stereotypes
11. Challenge and encourage clients to take action to prepare for and initiate role transitions by
    - Locating sources of relevant information and experience
    - Obtaining and interpreting information and experiences, and acquiring skills needed to make role transitions
12. Assist the client to acquire a set of employability and job search skills
13. Support and challenge clients to examine life-work roles, including the balance of work, leisure, family, and community in their careers

Individual/Group Assessment	Individual/group assessment skills considered essential for professionals engaging in career counseling. Demonstration of ability to

1. Assess personal characteristics such as aptitude, achievement, interests, values, and personality traits
2. Assess leisure interests, learning style, life roles, self-concept, career maturity, vocational identity, career indecision, work environment preference (e.g., work satisfaction), and other related life style/development issues

continued

Figure 1.2 *continued*

	3. Assess conditions of the work environment (such as tasks, expectations, norms, and qualities of the physical and social settings) 4. Evaluate and select valid and reliable instruments appropriate to the client's gender, sexual orientation, race, ethnicity, and physical and mental capacities 5. Use computer-delivered assessment measures effectively and appropriately 6. Select assessment techniques appropriate for group administration and those appropriate for individual administration 7. Administer, score, and report findings from career assessment instruments appropriately 8. Interpret data from assessment instruments and present the results to clients and to others 9. Assist the client and others designated by the client to interpret data from assessment instruments 10. Write an accurate report of assessment results
Information/Resources	Information/resource base and knowledge essential for professionals engaging in career counseling. Demonstration of knowledge of 1. Education, training, and employment trends; labor market information and resources that provide information about job tasks, functions, salaries, requirements, and future outlooks related to broad occupational fields and individual occupations 2. Resources and skills that clients utilize in life-work planning and management 3. Community/professional resources available to assist clients in career planning, including job search 4. Changing roles of women and men and the implications that this has for education, family, and leisure 5. Methods of good use of computer-based career information delivery systems (CIDS) and computer-assisted career guidance systems (CACGS) to assist with career planning
Program Promotion, Management, and Implementation	Knowledge and skills necessary to develop, plan, implement, and manage comprehensive career development programs in a variety of settings. Demonstration of knowledge of 1. Designs that can be used in the organization of career development programs 2. Needs assessment and evaluation techniques and practices 3. Organizational theories, including diagnosis, behavior, planning, organizational communication, and management useful in implementing and administering career development programs 4. Methods of forecasting, budgeting, planning, costing, policy analysis, resource allocation, and quality control 5. Leadership theories and approaches for evaluation and feedback, organizational change, decision making, and conflict resolution 6. Professional standards and criteria for career development programs 7. Societal trends and state and federal legislation that influence the development and implementation of career development programs

Figure 1.2 *continued*

	Demonstration of ability to

Demonstration of ability to

8. Implement individual and group programs in career development for specified populations
9. Train others in the appropriate use of computer-based systems for career information and planning.
10. Plan, organize, and manage a comprehensive career resource center
11. Implement career development programs in collaboration with others
12. Identify and evaluate staff competencies
13. Mount a marketing and public relations campaign in behalf of career development activities and services

Coaching, Consultation, and Performance Improvement

Knowledge and skills considered essential in relating to individuals and organizations that impact the career counseling and development process. Demonstration of ability to

1. Use consultation theories, strategies, and models
2. Establish and maintain a productive consultative relationship with people who can influence a client's career
3. Help the general public and legislators to understand the importance of career counseling, career development, and life-work planning
4. Impact public policy as it relates to career development and workforce planning
5. Analyze future organizational needs and current level of employee skills and develop performance improvement training
6. Mentor and coach employees

Diverse Populations

Knowledge and skills considered essential in relating to diverse populations that impact career counseling and development processes. Demonstration of ability to

1. Identify development models and multicultural counseling competencies
2. Identify developmental needs unique to various diverse populations, including those of different gender, sexual orientation, ethnic group, race, and physical or mental capacity
3. Define career development programs to accommodate needs unique to various diverse populations
4. Find appropriate methods or resources to communicate with individuals who have limited proficiency in English
5. Identify alternative approaches to meet career-planning needs for individuals of various diverse populations
6. Identify community resources and establish linkages to assist clients with specific needs
7. Assist other staff members, professionals, and community members in understanding the unique needs/characteristics of diverse populations with regard to career exploration, employment expectations, and economic/social issues
8. Advocate for the career development and employment of diverse populations
9. Design and deliver career development programs and materials to hard-to-reach populations

continued

Figure 1.2   *continued*

Supervision	Knowledge and skills considered essential in critically evaluating counselor or career development facilitator performance, maintaining and improving professional skills. Demonstration of

1. Ability to recognize own limitations as a career counselor and to seek supervision or refer clients when appropriate
2. Ability to utilize supervision on a regular basis to maintain and improve counselor skills
3. Ability to consult with supervisors and colleagues regarding client and counseling issues and issues related to one's own professional development as a career counselor
4. Knowledge of supervision models and theories
5. Ability to provide effective supervision to career counselors and career development facilitators at different levels of experience
6. Ability to provide effective supervision to career development facilitators at different levels of experience by
   - Knowledge of their roles, competencies, and ethical standards
   - Determining their competence in each of the areas included in their certification
   - Further training them in competencies, including interpretation of assessment instruments
   - Monitoring and mentoring their activities in support of the professional career counselor
   - Scheduling regular consultations for the purpose of reviewing their activities

Ethical/Legal Issues	Information base and knowledge essential for the ethical and legal practice of career counseling. Demonstration of knowledge of

1. Adherence to ethical codes and standards relevant to the profession of career counseling (e.g., NBCC, NCDA, and ACA)
2. Current ethical and legal issues that affect the practice of career counseling with all populations
3. Current ethical/legal issues with regard to the use of computer-assisted career guidance systems
4. Ethical standards relating to consultation issues
5. State and federal statutes relating to client confidentiality

Research/Evaluation	Knowledge and skills considered essential in understanding and conducting research and evaluation in career counseling and development. Demonstration of ability to

1. Write a research proposal
2. Use types of research and research designs appropriate to career counseling and development research
3. Convey research findings related to the effectiveness of career counseling programs
4. Design, conduct, and use the results of evaluation programs

Figure 1.2 *continued*	
	5. Design evaluation programs that take into account the need of various diverse populations, including persons of both genders, differing sexual orientations, different ethnic and racial backgrounds, and differing physical and mental capacities 6. Apply appropriate statistical procedures to career-development research
Technology	Knowledge and skills considered essential in using technology to assist individuals with career planning. Demonstration of knowledge of 1. Various computer-based guidance and information systems as well as services available on the Internet 2. Standards by which such systems and services are evaluated (e.g., NCDA and ACSCI) 3. Ways in which to use computer-based systems and Internet services that are consistent with ethical standards in order to assist individuals with career planning 4. Characteristics of clients that make them profit from use of technology-driven systems. 5. Methods to evaluate and select a system to meet local needs

ETHICS

Career professionals are likely to hold memberships in one or more organizations that dictate their on-the-job ethical behaviors. The ethical codes of each of these organizations require members to adhere to a certain standard of behavior regarding treatment of culturally diverse groups. These ethical codes have evolved to the point where they include greater and greater commitment to multiculturalism. The American Psychological Association (APA, 2002b) revised its ethical codes in 2002; the National Career Development Association (NCDA, 2003) did so in 2003; and the American Counseling Association (ACA, 2005) has made the most recent changes, in 2005. The issue of ethical behavior with diverse groups is addressed in each of these ethical codes. The codes for the ACA, APA, and NCDA may be found on the websites of the respective organizations.

The APA Ethical Principles of Psychologists and Code of Conduct 2002 (APA, 2002b) were generated in the same year as the APA Guidelines on Education, Training, Research, Practice, and Organizational Change for Psychologists. All psychologists, including vocational psychologists, are expected to adhere to both of these standards. Of the five basic Ethical Principles, two address issues of diversity: Justice (Principle D) and Respect for People's Rights and Dignity (Principle E). Principle D (Justice) states:

Psychologists recognize that fairness and justice entitle all persons to access to and benefit from the contributions of psychology and to equal quality in the processes, procedures and services being conducted by psychologists. Psychologists exercise reasonable judgment and take precautions to ensure that their potential biases, the boundaries of their competence, and the limitations of their expertise do not lead to or condone unjust practice (APA, 2002, p. 3–4).

Principle E (Respect for People's Rights and Dignity) states:

Psychologists respect the dignity and worth of all people and the rights of individuals to privacy, confidentiality, and self-determination. Psychologists are aware that special safeguards may be necessary to protect the rights and welfare of persons or communities whose vulnerabilities impair autonomous decision making. Psychologists are aware of and respect cultural, individual and role differences, including those based on age, gender, gender identity, race, ethnicity, culture, national origin, religion, sexual orientation, disability, language, and socioeconomic status and consider these factors when working with members of such groups. Psychologists try to eliminate the effect on their work of biases on those factors and they do not knowingly participate in or condone activities of others based upon such prejudices (APA, 2002, p. 4).

In addition to the above two specific principles, cultural issues are addressed throughout the code.

The new ACA Code of Ethics is even more visibly supportive of culturally sensitive behavior on the part of counselors than the APA Code. The preamble to the ACA Code states that "Association members recognize diversity, and embrace a cross-cultural approach in support of the worth, dignity, potential and uniqueness of people within their social context" (p. 3). Many of the statements in the Code regarding cultural sensitivity that had been buried in subsections of the previous ethical code have been moved to an introduction and to appropriate, more visible sections of the new Code. In addition subsections are devoted to work with multicultural and diversity considerations. Also, the new ACA Code of Ethics (2005) addresses at least one standard of appropriate behavior in multicultural career counseling.

The NCDA ethical codes are the least explicit of the three Codes regarding diversity standards, with only four specific references that apply. However, because the NCDA is a division of ACA, the ACA codes apply where no NCDA codes exist.

Over the years, the ethical codes of the above-named professional counseling organizations have all been severely criticized by multicultural authors because of the limited vision of counseling the codes have represented. The codes have reflected culturally encapsulated values that endorse a way of counseling that is individualistic, victim blaming, and responsive only to those that come from a background of privilege. It is ironic that to be culturally competent, counselors have had to violate their ethical codes when adherence to the codes may have been harmful to their clients.

For example, both APA and ACA have been criticized in the past for focusing on the individual to the exclusion of those from collectivist cultures. A unilateral rejection of dual relationships (counseling relationships that are both professional and personal) in the ethical codes of these organizations was imposed because of the belief that dual relationships always compromise the counseling relationship and cloud the objectivity of the counselor. However, subscribing to these codes has in the past created problems for counselors with clients from collectivist cultures who not only welcome helpers such as counselors into their families but also resent a counselor helping one individual to the exclusion of the rest of the family (Herlihy & Watson, 2003). The sterile approach of a person sitting in the counseling office and treating clients as if they were specimens in a laboratory is unacceptable in collectivist cultures. Further, several authors have suggested that dual relationships can be a good thing. Sometimes clients want such relationships because they prefer to share concerns with someone who is close to them and perhaps because objectivity is overrated (Sue, 1997; Parham, 1997; Herlihy & Watson, 2003). Also, for counselors working in some rural settings, dual relationships are unavoidable (Hedges, 1993; Herlihy & Corey, 1997), for instance on Native American reservations.

Another ethical issue that has been criticized in the past is the idea that bartering with clients is an unacceptable practice. Bartering has been clearly frowned upon by the ethical codes of the APA and ACA in the past. However, multicultural authors have suggested that in some areas of the county, individuals and families are too poor to pay in cash and are used to paying in kind by bartering. Moreover, gifts have been frowned upon by professional ethical codes, as they are seen to interfere with counseling objectivity. However, it is considered rude in some cultures to reject a gift (Sue, 2003) and impolite not to offer one.

It is heartening to see that both the APA and the ACA ethical guidelines now make provisions to bend the rules in cases in which doing so promotes cultural diversity. Because the ethical codes are now more responsive to cultural issues, counselors will be able to better meet the needs of all of their clients without feeling guilt or fear of possible sanctions for ethical violations.

Although the ACA Code of Ethics, 2005, addresses cultural issues in the introductions to the various sections of the code, the overall statement of the purpose to the code reads, "The introductions to each section discuss what counselors should aspire to with regard to ethical behavior and responsibility." This does cause some concern because not only are there statements in the introductions that were part of the previous, now outdated, code, but it also seems that rather than expecting counselors to engage in certain ethical behaviors, the code now indicates that such behaviors are considered only ideal. If this is the case, the ethical code has been weakened in regard to multicultural competence, even though the prominence of these competencies has increased. In contrast, the APA Ethical Principles state that "modifiers used in some of the standards of this Ethics Code (e.g., reasonably, appropriate, potentially) are included . . . when they would . . . eliminate injustice or inequality that would occur without the modifier. . . ." It would seem, therefore that the introduction to the APA code gives an opportunity to expand the application of the code to members of oppressed groups in the society. It is certain that these codes will continue to evolve and will continue to be responsive to the needs of diverse populations.

Unfortunately, ethical codes are simply guides for behavior rather than mandates. Rarely are they written in a manner that addresses every ethical issue that a counselor may encounter. As a result, counselors may find themselves in situations where they still have questions about the ethical and moral path to take. For career counselors to behave ethically, they first need to be knowledgeable of their professional organization's ethical codes. Ethical codes have traditionally been designed to provide minimum standards for professional behavior in a particular field. Typically, adherence to the ethical guidelines leads to behavior that exceeds legal requirements. When counselors face questions that do not have clear answers in the ethical guidelines, however, they should always discuss the problem with a professional of like qualifications and membership in the same professional organization who is also knowledgeable about the current code of ethics. If for any reason the counselor is still unsure about the appropriate action, further consultation with another professional or consultation with the professional organization itself would be the best course.

Four career counseling ethical dilemmas are presented below. Following each dilemma are the applicable ethical codes from ACA, APA, and NCDA. Suggestions will then be made as to how counselors should proceed if they or someone else is in violation of an ethical code.

Dilemma 1

Caroline is a thirty-four-year-old white female employment counselor whose lesbian client is in search of a position in an organization that will let her claim her partner on her insurance and as a beneficiary on her retirement. Caroline believes that the client has unrealistic expectations and gently breaks this news to her client. Unfortunately, the client is adamant about finding a company that will provide these benefits. Caroline is baffled because (a) the client has not even received a job offer from anyone, and (b) even if she does receive an offer, no one is going to allow her to claim her same-sex partner. Caroline decides that perhaps a lesbian counselor would be able to talk some sense into this client. She makes plans to refer the client to another counselor and will break the news to the client in the next session.

The codes referenced for this dilemma refer to Section A of the ACA Code of Ethics (A1.3, A4.b, A6.a, A11.a, A11.b); Standard 2: Competence of the APA Ethical Principles and Code of Conduct (2.01b) and Section A: General and Section B: The Counseling Relationship in the NCDA Ethical Standards (A.10; B11; B13).

Caroline's dilemma, it seems, has more to do with her biases toward lesbian clients than it has to do with her competence. She would have been acting ethically if her only reason for the referral were that she didn't have the competence to work with the client's problem. However, that doesn't seem to be the case here. A more ethical course of action for Caroline would have been to consult with her colleague on how to proceed with her lesbian client. In that case, she may have discovered that many companies do in fact offer same-sex partner benefits. As it is, she seems to be avoiding facing her homophobia or learning how to handle a situation with a gay or lesbian theme.

Dilemma 2

Brian is a fifty-six-year-old African American male employee assistance counselor who has been assigned a large number of clients who have recently been displaced from their jobs. They will each receive six weeks of severance pay as well as six sessions of career counseling to help them find a new job. Most of the clients are Latinos or Latinas and Native Americans—both males and females. Because the task is so overwhelming, he decides to maximize his time and minimize his effort on individual cases. He has recently completed a workshop on how to do group interpretations of a career inventory, so he will give all the clients an interest inventory and a personality inventory to take home and complete. Because the group is diverse, he feels he should know where they stand in terms of ability, so he will administer a paper and pencil intelligence test at the first session. Brian will call the group back together when the results from all the testing come in and provide a group interpretation of the interest inventory, personality inventory, and intelligence test. He will follow up with any individuals who just don't get it.

This dilemma involves Section E: Evaluation and Assessment of the ACA Code of Ethics (E.2a, E.2b, E.3.a, E.6.c, E.8, E.9.a); Standard 2: Competence (2.01b) and Standard 9: Assessment (9.02b, 9.02b, 9.06, 9.09c) of the APA; and Section B (B.1, B.13) and C (C.1, C.12) of the NCDA Ethical Standards.

Brian should be applauded for his efficiency. However, such efficiency can get him into a great deal of trouble ethically. The ethical codes cited above have to do with his knowledge of diverse cultures and his competence and knowledge of assessment. Because his clients come from diverse groups, each client will have different characteristics, influenced by culture and acculturation, which affect career development. Brian needs to take the time to work with each client in an initial session to assess his or her cultural identity and career problems. Then perhaps he can screen each client for group counseling and assess the feasibility of group interpretation. Blanket administration without first working with clients on an individual basis is unethical according to all three ethical codes. Finally, a group assessment must also be done with cautions that Brian, it appears, does not plan to take.

Dilemma 3

Isabel, a twenty-year-old Puerto Rican college student, has been referred by her mother to Maria, a career counselor at her college. Maria and Isabel's mother were college roommates, so Isabel's mother is grateful that a close family friend whom she trusts completely can help her daughter make a major life decision regarding her future career. Maria is happy to see Isabel, and after they have worked together for a few weeks, Maria receives an invitation from Isabel to attend a family gathering. Isabel says that her mother wants to use this occasion to thank Maria for all her work with her daughter. Isabel is most anxious for Maria to come and will not take no for an answer. Maria agrees to go but first discusses confidentiality again with Isabel. Maria reminds Isabel that it is her intent to respect Isabel's wishes as to what to tell her family about the counseling process and what not to tell.

Maria's dilemma involves ACA Code of Ethics Section A: The Counseling Relationship and B: Confidentiality, Privileged Communication (A.5.c, A.5.d, B.1.a, B.1.c); APA Ethical Principles and Code of Conduct Standard 3: Human Relations and 4: Privacy and Confidentiality (3.05a 3.05b, 4.01, 4.05a); and NCDA's Ethical Standard B: Counseling Relationship (B1, B2).

As discussed earlier in this chapter, the prohibition on participating in social events with clients was a subject in the ethical codes that was criticized in the past because of the limits it placed on culturally different populations, who expect such interactions. Maria seems to have given consideration to what would and would not be beneficial to her client and has decided that it would be more beneficial to attend the function than to refuse the invitation. She is aware that the parents may want to pump her for information, so Maria appropriately discusses this issue with her client before agreeing to attend the celebration.

Dilemma 4

Jessie is an African American career counselor who is new to a community agency that serves a Native American population. Jessie is proud of her multicultural training, and, though she has never worked with Native Americans before, she feels confident that she can do the job. Her twenty-two-year-old client, who is a mother of two, has been delightful to work with. However, the time has come for the client to make some decisions, and she seems very hesitant. She says she would like to bring in family members to help her out with the decision. Jessie is happy to do so and encourages her client to bring in her family. Jessie has not received training in family therapy but she has consulted with family members before. Also, this will not be a family therapy session, so Jessie is certain that she will be able to work well with them.

The ACA codes involved in this case include Section A: The Counseling Relationship (A.2.c, A.5.e, A7) and C: Professional Responsibility (C.2.a, C.2.b); APA Standard 2: Competence (2.01a, 2.01b, 2.01c) and NCDA Ethical Standard A: General (A.7).

Jessie is to be applauded for her eagerness to work with a population with which she is not totally familiar. However, the ethical codes governing her behavior have to do with competence, knowledge of cultural groups, and professional responsibilities. It would have been better if Jessie had discussed her plan with her supervisor and had included the supervisor in the family session.

For the purpose of discussion, assume that the counselors in the above dilemmas did not seek advice from anyone regarding the ethics of their behaviors. If any of the counselors' behaviors have, in fact, been unethical, colleagues are required to take action. Typically, most organizations will try to resolve ethical violations informally within the organization. The counselors will gather to discuss the dilemma and take whatever action is necessary to resolve it. However, if a client has been harmed, an informal handling of the situation is probably not an option, and the counselor will be brought before the organization's ethics committee.

As the above scenarios have illustrated, competence in multicultural career counseling is a strong safety net for behaving ethically. Although there is no guarantee that counselors will always avoid an ethical dilemma, the best advice for any professional is always to discuss the behavior with a supervisor or knowledgeable colleague prior to engaging in questionable actions (ACA, 2005).

SYNTHESIZING MULTICULTURAL COMPETENCIES AND CAREER COUNSELING COMPETENCIES

Neither the AMCD nor the NCDA statements assist the counselor in synthesizing the two sets of competencies: multicultural competencies and career counseling competencies. Ward and Bingham (1993) offered ideas for synthesizing these skills through a multicultural career counseling checklist. The checklist includes categories in which counselors identify their awareness and knowledge of the following areas: counselor preparation, exploration and assessment, negotiation, and working consensus. Although it is an excellent start, the checklist leaves out several of the career counseling competencies described earlier in this chapter and focuses mostly on knowledge of the client's culture and world view. Unearthing the compatibilities between the two sets of competencies will be helpful when combining them. The goal of this book is to facilitate this synthesis so that you will become a multiculturally competent career counselor.

The multicultural competencies will be covered in more detail in Chapter 2, "Awareness of Your Own Cultural Heritage"; Chapter 3, "Awareness of Your Own Values, Biases, and Prejudices," and Chapter 4, "Awareness of Clients' Worldview." Chapter 4 will also cover one of the career counseling competencies, "Diverse Populations." To gain multicultural competence, it is very important to have done the work in these three chapters before moving ahead to the rest of the book.

The second part of the book, will apply the multicultural competencies to the career counseling competencies as follows: Chapter 5, "Using Career Theories as a Map," covers the career theories and their appropriate application in multicultural career counseling. Chapter 6, "Individual and Group Counseling Skills," addresses the skills considered essential for culturally effective career counseling; Chapter 7, "Testing and Assessment," reviews appropriate use of testing with multicultural populations, and Chapter 8, "Social Action," provides information on extending commitment to cultural competence by advocating for clients against social injustices.

REFERENCES

American Counseling Association (2005). ACA Code of Ethics 2005. Retrieved November 21, 2006 from *http://www.counseling.org/Resources/CodeOfEthics/TP/Home/CT2.aspx*

American Psychological Association (2002a). Guidelines and principles for accreditation of programs in professional psychology. Retrieved November 21, 2006 from *www.apa.org/ed/G&P2.pdf.*

American Psychological Association (2002b). Ethical principles of psychologists and code of conduct. Retrieved November 21, 2006 from *www.apa.org/ethics/code2002.pdf*

Arredondo, P., & Perez, P. (2003). Expanding multicultural competence through social justice leadership. *Counseling Psychologist, 31,* 282–289.

Arredondo, P., Toporek, R., Brown, S. P., Jones, J., Locke, D. C., Sanchez, J., & Stadler, H. (1996). Operationalization of the multicultural counseling competencies. *Journal of Multicultural Counseling and Development, 24,* 42–78.

Burkard. A., Knox, S., Groen, M., Perez, M., & Hess, S. (2006). European American therapist self-disclosure in cross-cultural counseling. *Journal of Counseling Psychology, 53,* 15–25.

Council for the Accreditation of Counseling and Related Educational Programs (2001). 2001 standard. *www.cacrep.org/2001standards.html* Retrieved November 21, 2006.

Das, A. K. (1995). Rethinking multicultural counseling: Implications for counselor education. *Journal of Counseling and Development, 74,* 45–52.

Engels, D. W., Minor, C. W., Sampson, J. P., & Splete, H. H. (1995). Career counseling specialty: History, development, and prospect. *Journal of Counseling and Development, 74,* 134–138.

Evans, K. M., & Larrabee, M. J. (2002). Teaching the multicultural counseling competencies and revised career counseling competencies simultaneously. *Journal of Multicultural Counseling and Development, 30,* 21–39.

Evans, K. M., & Rotter, J. C. (2000). Multicultural family approaches to career counseling. *The Family Journal, 8,* 67–71.

Falicov, C. J. (1995). Training to think culturally: A multidimensional comparative framework. *Family Process, 34,* 363–388.

Hedges, L. (1993, July/August). In praise of dual relatiohsips. Part II: Essential dual relatedness in developmental psychotherapy. *The California Therapist,* pp. 42–46.

Herlihy, B., & Corey, G. (1997). *Boundary issues in counseling.* Alexandria, VA: American Counseling Association.

Herlihy, B., & Watson, Z. E. (2003). Ethical issues and multicultural competence in counseling. In D. Harper and J. McFadden (Eds.), *Culture and counseling: New approaches* (pp. 363–378). Boston: Allyn & Bacon.

Herr, E. L., Cramer, S. H., & Niles, S. G. (2004). *Career guidance and counseling through the lifespan: Systematic approaches.* Boston: Pearson Education, Inc.

Maxie, A., Arnold, D., & Stephenson, M. (2006). Do therapists address ethnic and racial differences in cross-cultural psychotherapy? *Psychotherapy: Theory, Research, Practice, Training, 43,* 85–98.

NCDA (author), (2003). National Career Development Association Ethical Standards (Revised 2003) *http://www.ncda.org/pdf/EthicalStandards.pdf* (Retrieved November 21, 2006)

NCDA (author). 1997. Career Counseling Competencies. (www.ncda.org/pdf/counselingcompetencies.pdf). Retrieved August 28, 2006.

Parham, T. A. (1997). An African-centered view of dual relationships. In B. Herlihy & G. Corey (Eds.), *Boundary issues in counseling* (pp. 109–111). Alexandria, VA: American Counseling Association.

Pedersen, P. B. (1984). Levels of intercultural communication using the Rehearsal Demonstration model, *Journal of Non-White Concerns in Personnel & Guidance, 12*(2), 57–68.

Ponterotto, J. G. (1997). Multicultural counseling training: A competency model and national survey. In D. B. Pope-Davis & H. L. K. Coleman (Eds.), *Multicultural counseling competencies: Assessment, education, and training, and supervision.* (pp. 111–130). Thousand Oaks, CA: Sage Publications.

Ponterotto, J. G., Fuertes, J. N., & Chen, E. C. (2000). Models of multicultural counseling. In S. D. Brown & R. W. Lent (Eds.) *Handbook of counseling psychology* (3rd ed.) (pp. 639–669). Hoboken, NJ: John Wiley & Sons, Inc.

Ridley, C. R., Espelage, D. L., & Rubinstein, K. J. (1997). Course development in multicultural counseling. In D. B. Pope-Davis & H. L. K. Coleman (Eds.), *Multicultural counseling competencies: Assessment, education, and training, and supervision.* (pp. 131–158). Thousand Oaks, CA: Sage Publications.

Roysircar, G., Sandhu, D. S., & Bibbins, V. E. Sr. (Eds.) (2003). *Multicultural competencies: A guidebook of practices.* Alexandria, VA: Association for Multicultural Counseling & Development.

Sue, D. W. (1997). Multicultural perspectives on multiple relationships. In B. Herlihy & G. Corey (Eds.), *Boundary issues in counseling* (pp. 106–109). Alexandria, VA: American Counseling Association.

Sue, D. W. (2003). *Overcoming racism: The journey to liberation.* San Francisco: Jossey-Bass.

Sue, D. W., Bernier, J. B., Durran, M., Feinberg, L., Pedersen, P., Smith, E., & Vasques-Nuttall, E. (1982). Position paper: Cross-cultural counseling competencies. *Counseling Psychologist, 10,* 45–52.

Sue, D., Arredondo, P., & McDavis, R. J. (1992). Multicultural competencies/standards: A pressing need. *Journal of Counseling and Development, 70*(4), 477–486.

Sue, D. W., Carter, R. T., Casas, J. M., Fouad, A., Ivey, A. E., Jensen, M., LaFromboise, T., Manese, J. E., Ponterotto, J. G., & Vazquez-Nutall, E. (1998). *Multicultural counseling competencies: Individual and organizational development.* Thousand Oaks, CA: Sage Publications.

Thompson, C. E. F., & Jenal, S. T. (1994). Interracial and intraracial quasi-counseling interaction when counselors avoid discussing race. *Journal of Counseling and Development, 41,* 484–491.

Tomlinson-Clark, S., & Wang, V. O. (1999). A paradigm for racial-cultural training in the development of counselor cultural competencies. In M. S. Kiselica (Ed.) *Prejudice and racism during multicultural training.* Alexandria, VA: American Counseling Association.

Vera, E. M., & Speight, S. L. (2003). Multicultural competence, social justice, and counseling psychology: Expanding our roles. *Counseling Psychologist, 31*(3), 253–272.

Ward, C. M., & Bingham, R. P. (1993). Career assessment of ethnic minority women. *Journal of Career Assessment, 1,* 246–257.

CHAPTER 2
Awareness of Your Own Cultural Heritage

My professor just told us we would have to write a paper on our own culture, and I panicked. I don't believe that I have a culture. My family tree has people form Scotland, Ireland, Norway, Sweden, England, and Hungary. But all of that is so far back in the family history; no one has bothered to hold on to the cultures of these different national-ities. I feel like my culture is like Heinz 57 varieties and I don't have a clue where to begin. How do I write a paper on my culture if it doesn't exist?

—An entry from a student's journal

It is not unusual for counselors in training to write an entry like the one above when confronted with the task of defining their own culture. More often than not, the writer of such an entry will be a European American, who does not identify with any specific white ethnic group (Irish, Italian, German, and so forth). These individuals claim that they have no culture because they have confused ethnicity with culture, which is very understandable. Culture is very complex, and definitions of culture run from narrow to broad. Narrowly defined, culture is limited to ethnicity, language, ideology, nationality, and religion. Pedersen (1999) offers his broad definition of culture: "the total way of life of a people including their interpersonal relations as well as their attitudes" (p. 7). Similarly, Arredondo and colleagues (1996) define culture as "patterns of learned thinking and behavior of people communicated across generations through traditions, language, and artifacts." (p. 40). Pedersen (1999) also states that broader definitions of culture are becoming more accepted and provide for greater application of culture to all counseling relationships.

Once culture has been adequately defined, it does not take long for former culture-less students to feel comfortable exploring their own culture. Investigation of one's culture involves identifying with the common language, history, philosophy of life, traditions, concept of family and kinship, work, governance, education, communication styles, and religion of one's group. It also involves exploring demographic variables such as gender, age, geography, and socioeconomic status.

Several authors have pointed out that all cultures are learned, shared, and dynamic (Gollnick & Chinn, 1994; Pedersen, 1994, 1999). Culture must be taught to others in order to survive; more than one person or family must adhere to the beliefs and traditions; and culture must change and adapt as the world changes. Cultural lessons begin in childhood when children are socialized to the norms of the culture in which they live (Gollnick & Chinn, 1994). Children learn the language, cultural policies, appropriate behavior, roles and expectations, sex roles, and acceptable occupations for their culture. These lessons come from family members, family friends, teachers, clergy, and other powerful adults (Gollnick & Chinn, 1994).

Cultural learning begins at an early age and continues until adulthood. Our cultural values, beliefs, behaviors, and so forth are natural to us after years of training (Gollnick & Chinn 1994). The lessons become internalized to the point where "we often confuse biological and cultural heritage" (pp. 6–9). This confusion has led to debates as to whether psychological and other characteristics such as intelligence are the result of nature (biological) or nurture (social/environmental). Such debates will continue, but it is important for counselors to remember that everyone is socialized into a culture. Gollnick and Chinn call this process enculturation. Though our culture defines a great part of our identity, it does not influence our genetic makeup.

Because we internalize our culture so completely, we are often unaware of cultural influences in our lives—much like the student who made the journal entry that began this chapter. There are a number of activities included in this chapter that may be helpful to anyone who is doubtful about his or her cultural heritage. These exercises are designed to help individuals discover that they do indeed have a culture.

Exercises for Unearthing Your Culture

Exercise 1: A Different World

This is an imagery exercise that should be done in a quiet spot where you will not be interrupted. Begin by taking two or three deep breaths—inhaling through your nose and exhaling through your mouth. Relax your body and clear your mind of all extraneous thoughts. Have someone read or record the instructions for this visualization.

Imagine that when you woke up this morning, you were in a different world. In this world, no one looks like or you speaks your language. None of the foods you like are available. In fact, you don't even recognize the food that you have been given. The rituals the people practice (you think the rituals may be religious) are completely foreign, as are the strange ways the people move their faces to express emotions. Their manner of speaking seems hostile and rude to you.

What will you miss most from your old world while living in this new world? Write your thoughts in the spaces below:

_____

_____

_____

_____

_____

_____

For many, this imagery exercise is one of the quickest and easiest ways to recognize one's culture. Many counselors find that the exercise helps them to get a better understanding of the importance of their way of life. They also realize that there are others whose way of life may differ and whose values, expectations, and traditions may seem strange to them. As such, it helps them develop empathy for those who are not members of their own cultural group.

Exercise 2: Recording Values and Traditions

Write an essay, or videotape a message to your children or to young people in your family. Discuss what you learned from your family and significant adults in your culture about race, gender, religion, traditions, traditional food, your geographic region, education, sexual orientation, manners, socioeconomic status, and powerful individuals. In addition, you may want to write about the origins of your family history in the United States. If your family immigrated—what was the immigration like, how did they adjust to the United States? If writing rather than videotaping, use the spaces below for your response.

_____

_____

_____

_____

_____

_____

Exercise 3: A Cultural Investigation

A very fruitful strategy for exploring your own culture is to investigate it as if you are from a different culture from your own. McGrath and Axelson (1999) and Parker (1998) recommend a cultural interview in which you ask people who identify as members of your culture specific questions about its characteristics. McGrath and Axelson as well as Haley (1990) suggest you start by interviewing your oldest relative. You will need to tease out characteristics that are representative of the whole culture as opposed to those characteristics that are unique to your own family. Here are some questions that you may want to include. (Questions are adapted from McGrath and Axelson, 1999, p. 52.)

(a) How would you describe your family culture?

_____

_____

(b) Is the traditional culture still intact or has it changed greatly? How?

_____

_____

(c) Is there still a cultural community?

_____

_____

(d) What occupations did your ancestors hold? Are those occupational choices typical of your culture?

_____

_____

(e) What are your family's attitudes toward work and vocation? What are their attitudes toward the culture?

_____

_____

After the interview is over, reflect on it by answering the following questions of yourself. (Questions adapted from McGrath and Axelson, 1999, p. 52.)

(a) Are you living up to your family of origin's expectations? How or how not?

_____

_____

(b) Are you living up to your family's culture's expectations? How or how not?

_____

_____

(c) What do you think a person of another culture (pick one) would think of your culture as you have "discovered" it? (p. 53)

_____

_____

THE DOMINANT AMERICAN CULTURE

The diverse groups that have immigrated to the United States during its history have all been expected to leave behind the cultures from their countries of origin and adopt an "American" culture common to all. This "melting pot" metaphor was prevalent for most of the history of the United States. However, the metaphor became more problematic during and after the civil rights movement when the world could see that all Americans were not included in the melting pot, that in fact the American landscape was more akin to a "salad" or a "mosaic" of different parts existing side by side than to a blended melting pot. Initially, those Americans who were visibly different from the dominant group were, more often than not, legally forbidden to blend in with others. For example, prior to Civil Rights legislation, there were laws in many of the Southeastern states that segregated people of color (most specifically, African Americans) from whites in public places. People of color were also legally forbidden to marry whites in many states. This type of separation limited the exposure of whites to other racial and cultural groups. However, members of these visibly different groups (African Americans, Asian Americans, Hispanics, and American Indians) were still exposed to the dominant U.S. culture.

Following the definitions of culture outlined earlier in this chapter, the dominant U.S. culture can be characterized as follows: the predominant language is English, the government is a republic, the family is nuclear, religion is Christianity (though citizens practice it a myriad of different ways), basic education (K–12) is free, "American" foods are hot dogs (or hamburgers) and apple pie, the predominant socioeconomic group is the middle class, and the most prized values are rugged individualism and the belief in meritocracy. Everyone who lives in the United States is familiar with these cultural elements, and certainly those who were born in the United States have internalized these elements. However, other cultural groups may value languages different from English, believe in the extended family, prefer other foods, be predominantly from the lower classes, and/or believe in collectivism (valuing the group over the individual). How much an individual internalizes the U.S. culture is dependent on the individual, the number of years the person has lived in the United States, the strength of the individual's other cultural characteristics (from the person's country of origin, or cultural or racial group), and the consequences for adopting U.S. culture (rewards or punishments).

A person is said to be acculturated if he or she "identifies with the attitudes, behaviors, and values of the predominant macroculture" (Lee, 1995, p. 12). The more an individual's own acculturation exceeds or lags behind that of his or her family, the more conflict there is, and the more isolated the individual may become. At the same time, the more an individual resembles people from the dominant cultural group (middle class, Protestant, European Americans), the more likely it is that he or she will enjoy a privileged status in society. In other words, U.S. society is geared toward meeting the needs and desires of the dominant group to the extent that the dominant group has unearned advantages. A more in-depth discussion of privilege occurs in a later chapter in this text.

The dominant U.S. culture is like an umbrella that covers all the other cultural groups in the country. It is important, therefore, to have an understanding of dominant U.S. culture, because it has undoubtedly been intertwined into the internal culture of many people—career counselors and their clients included.

CULTURAL RELATIVISM AND WORLDVIEW

Two critical concepts have emerged from the study of multicultural counseling. The first is "cultural relativism" and the second is "worldview."

Cultural Relativism

Cultural relativism is the belief that everything is subjective and that nothing can be considered outside of the context in which it exists (Ridley et al., 2001). In other words, we must always take into account a person's culture when we observe any behavior. For example, let's consider what it means to be suspicious of someone. To be suspicious of someone means different things in different cultures, and at the same time it also means different things to individuals who are members of the same culture. A member of an oppressed group (such as American Indians) may distrust or may be suspicious of anyone outside that group. However, specific Indian tribes may be accepting of selected non-Indians. In cultural relativism, the context is the primary consideration. While cultural relativism has been criticized by some as being too broad a concept to be useful in counseling, it sets the stage for counselors to consider not only the differences among groups but also the differences within groups.

Worldview

The concept of worldview has become a staple in multicultural training and counseling. Essentially, "worldview" denotes one's beliefs about the world and one's relationship to the world. Sire's (1976) definition of worldview is "the presuppositions and assumptions we hold about our world" (p. 17). Sue and Sue (2003) suggest that worldview is inclusive of cultural factors such as values, expectations, and so forth, but also includes personal factors such as thoughts, attitudes, and behaviors. In other words, worldview is shaped by cultural socialization (in which we learn acceptable behavior, beliefs, and attitudes) as well as personal experiences and the meaning people take from those experiences. If we want to understand others, we not only need to understand the worldviews of others, but we also have to understand our own worldview.

Locus of Control/Responsibility

D. W. Sue (1978) and Sue and Sue (2003) describe individual worldviews via two cognitive concepts that are independent of one another—locus of control and locus of responsibility. According to Sue and Sue, locus of control and locus of responsibility can be either internal or external. Individuals with an internal locus of control believe that they have control over themselves and their behaviors while individuals with an external locus of control believe that outside forces, such as luck and fate, control their beliefs and behaviors. Individuals with an internal locus of responsibility are likely to claim responsibility for their actions while individuals with an external sense of responsibility are likely to place blame on others for their actions.

Figure 2.1 Locus of Control/Responsibility: The Four Quadrants

Quadrant 1—An individual with an internal locus of control and an internal locus of responsibility would say, "I'm okay and the system is okay" (Axelson, 1999). Sue and Sue (2003) state that this worldview represents the dominant European American perspective.

Quandrant 2—Individuals with an external locus of control and an internal locus of responsibility are people who feel marginalized because they believe in the dominant culture's view of things and at the same time blame themselves and those within their own cultural group for not realizing the American Dream.

Quadrant 3—Individuals with an external locus of control and an external locus of responsibility would say, "I'm not okay, and society is not okay" (Axelson, 1999). According to Sue and Sue (2003) individuals in this quadrant have acquired a learned helplessness perspective. These individuals believe that they are not in control of what happens in their lives and that they are not responsible for what happens to them either. They believe that the barriers that have been erected to keep them from succeeding are too difficult to break down, so they give up.

Quadrant 4—Individuals with an internal locus of control and an external locus of responsibility are the healthiest of minority individuals in terms of worldview. These individuals believe that they are okay, but the system is not (Axelson, 1999). These individuals know that they have control over their own behaviors and beliefs, but they also know that there are forces beyond their control that are responsible for some of their problems. Racism and discrimination are real to these individuals, but they do not internalize negative impressions of their racial or cultural group.

		LOCUS OF RESPONSIBILITY	
		INTERNAL	EXTERNAL
L O C U S **O F** **C O N T R O L**	INTERNAL	Quadrant 1 *Internal* locus of control and *internal* locus of responsibility	Quadrant 4 *Internal* locus of control and *external* locus of responsibility
	EXTERNAL	Quadrant 2 *External* locus of control and *internal* locus of responsibility	Quadrant 3 *External* locus of control and *external* locus of responsibility

Adapted from Eliminating cultural oppression in counseling: Toward a general theory by D. W. Sue, 1978, *Journal of Counseling Psychology*, 25, p. 422. Copyright by the *Journal of Counseling Psychology*.

Sue and Sue have placed these orientations into a four-quadrant model, as illustrated in Figure 2.1, which shows how these orientations intersect with one another. Each of the four quadrants demonstrates a different worldview, one of which is characteristic of the dominant European American perspective and the other three of which are characteristic of minority group perspectives.

Locus of Control/Responsibility Exercise

In which quadrant of the locus of control/responsibility model do you place yourself? Why specifically do you place yourself in this quadrant?

_____

_____

_____

Value Orientation

Although Sue and Sue's four quadrant locus of control/responsibility model is a helpful way of understanding worldview, worldview is a dynamic concept that has changed since Sue's original focus on the differences between groups. More recently, differences within groups have been explored in more depth (Ibrahim, 1991; Myers et al., 1991). A major reason for the shift was to keep counselors from developing stereotypes of their clients as completely subject to their groups and to help counselors better empathize with their clients' individual worldviews (Trevino, 1996).

For instance, in 1961 Kluckhohn and Strodtbeck began a study that compared the cultural values of five diverse groups in the United States. The groups were the Navaho Indians, Spanish Americans, Texas homesteaders, Zuni (Pueblo) Indians, and Mormons. As a result of this intensive ten-year study, Kluckhohn and Strodtbeck (1961) found differences in five value orientations: human nature, human activity, time orientation, social relationships, and relationship to nature. Each of these value orientations was broken into three possible viewpoints. For time orientation the viewpoints were past, present, and future; for human activity, the viewpoints were being, being-in-becoming, and doing; for social relationships the viewpoints were linear, collateral, and individualistic; for relationship with nature, the viewpoints were subjugation, harmony, and mastery over; and for human nature, the viewpoints were that people were inherently good, bad, or neutral. Different cultural groups weighed in differently on each of value orientations and viewpoints. For example, Sue and Sue (2003) noted that while Puerto Ricans typically value a present time focus, European Americans value a future time focus. The dominant European American view of activity leaned toward doing, while other cultures valued just being. Ibrahim (1991) applied to counseling the value orientations and viewpoints from Kluckhohn and Strodtbeck's study to create a multicultural counseling assessment instrument. According to Ibrahim, the different viewpoints within the value orientations can lead to conflict in counseling situations. Therefore, it is important for counselors to identify the cultural values they adhere to and those they reject. Further, if counselors reject any of their own group's cultural values, this may influence counseling situations in which the client is someone from the same culture but does not reject that value. To assist counselors in determining their worldview and to help counselors determine the worldview of their clients, Ibrahim and Kahn (1984, 1987) developed the Scale to Assess Worldview. Ibrahim and Kahn (1987) describe their scale as one that assesses "beliefs, values, and assumptions on . . . views of human nature, interpersonal relationships, nature, time, and activity" (p. 163). An individual rates his or her level of agreement with an item on a scale of 1–5 (strongly agree to strongly disagree). The authors supply the following example of an item in their journal article:

Human beings are a combination of good and evil.

Strongly Disagree			Strongly Agree	
1	2	3	4	5 (p. 167)

In terms of career counseling, it is important to remember that value orientation in terms of work situations varies from one culture to the next. European Americans, African Americans and Asian Americans all value the "doing" orientation of human activity. European Americans value doing for individual achievement of success, Asian Americans value doing that achieves honor and fulfills family and cultural expectations, and African Americans value doing activities that overcome barriers to achieving success (Sue & Sue, 2003). On the other hand, American Indians and Latinos value the being-in-becoming orientation of human activity. This means that they believe that doing is not as important as living in harmony with the universe, achieving serenity, and valuing individuals for existing (being), not for what they have achieved. Understanding one's own worldview as well as that of others is an essential skill for a culturally competent counselor.

You may wish to complete the following exercise, which utilizes Kluckhohn and Strodtbeck's value orientations, to examine your worldview more closely.

Value Orientations: One-Minute Papers

This is an exercise that can help you understand your worldview. Write a brief essay on each of the topics listed below. Spend no more than one minute writing each essay.

(a) What is your view of human nature? Are people innately good, bad, neutral? Explain why.

_____

_____

_____

_____

_____

(b) What is your most valued human activity (doing, being-in-becoming, or self-growth)?

_____

_____

_____

_____

_____

(c) From what point of view do you focus on time? Is it more important to focus on the past and learn from history? Or is it more important to enjoy the moment that you are in rather than the past or future? Or is it more important to look to the future and plan for a better tomorrow?

_____

_____

_____

_____

_____

_____

(d) What do you believe is the best relationship between humans and nature? Should humans try to assert power over nature and control it? Should people live in harmony with nature? Or should humans accept the fact that they have no control over nature?

_____

_____

_____

_____

_____

(e) What should relationships among humans be like? Should they be linear (some people lead others)? Or should they be collateral (meaning that groups should work together to solve problems)? Or should they be individualistic (meaning that each person should be self-sufficient and stand on his or her own two feet)?

_____

_____

_____

_____

_____

Similarly, Pedersen (1994) co-designed a sophisticated model for understanding worldview—the Interpersonal Cultural Grid (Hines & Pedersen, 1980). The Intrapersonal Cultural Grid provides a way to assess "an individual's personal-cultural orientation in a particular situation through attention to his or her behavior and its meaning" (p. 135). The following exercises utilizes Pedersen's intrapersonal cultural grid in assessing worldview.

Using the Intrapersonal Cultural Grid

Using Pederson's intrapersonal cultural grid, you will be able to plot your personal-cultural orientation by examining social system variables such as nationality, religion, social status, and affiliations with others, as well as other variables, such as gender, age, and physical ability.

Step 1. Choose an activity that you wish to analyze such as writing a letter of application for a job. Describe in detail how you would go about writing that letter.

_____

_____

Step 2. Identify the outcomes you expect from this activity. For example, you may expect to write a letter that will be good enough to get you a job, that will represent you in a good light, that will keep your name in circulation, or that will help you move forward in your career.

_____

_____

_____

_____

Step 3. Explore the personal values that accompany your expectations such as valuing yourself as an employee, recognizing your own achievements, and appreciating your own abilities.

_____

_____

_____

_____

Step 4. Examine the origins of these values. Did you get them from your family, your culture, your experience, etc? If your letter reflects certain values, for instance, doing a job well or working hard, where do these values come from—your family and culture, your experiences, or some other source? Pedersen indicates that investigating the origins of your own values when doing a particular activity reflects your own enculturation and socialization.

_____

_____

_____

_____

Unfortunately, many of the skills traditionally taught in counseling programs don't take into account multiple worldviews, and this lack of adjustment for different cultures may be the cause of premature termination of ethnic minority clients (Sue & Sue, 2003). More about the worldviews of specific groups will be addressed in Chapter 4. A very important part of one's worldview is one's racial/cultural identity, which is considered in the next section.

RACIAL/CULTURAL IDENTITY DEVELOPMENT MODELS

As mentioned earlier, one criticism of multicultural sensitivity training has been that counselors end up failing to appreciate the differences between individuals from the same ethnic minority group. They might erroneously conclude that every individual within a particular group has similar experiences, expectations, values, beliefs, and behaviors. More recently, Sue and Sue (2003) have credited both their own and other newer racial/cultural identity development models (which will be discussed in more detail below) with helping counselors to acknowledge and recognize within-group differences among ethnic minority groups. Sue and Sue also state that counselor knowledge of racial/cultural identity development models helps to decrease premature termination of counseling by racial/cultural minority clients because counselors are more aware of possible client reactions to counseling. Therefore, counselors can offer intervention strategies that are more appropriate to the client's particular stage of racial/cultural identity development. Sue and Sue point out that racial identity models acknowledge the "sociopolitical influences in shaping minority identity . . . [incorporating] the effects of racism and prejudice [oppression] upon the identity transformation of their victims" (p. 208).

In addition to helping counselors understand their clients better, racial/cultural identity development models provide counselors with a theoretical framework for understanding their own racism, prejudice, and privilege. The goal of multicultural education is essentially to assist counselors in developing a positive racial/cultural identity of their own. A positive racial/cultural identity entails valuing one's own race without making denigrating comparisons between one's own race and that of others (Helms, 1984).

Racial/cultural identity theories helped to explain racism from the "target's" perspective. "Target" is the term used by social psychologists to describe those groups who are targets for prejudice and racism (Swim, Cohen & Hyers, 1998). William Cross (1971) was one of the pioneers of racial/cultural identity theory building, and in his article entitled "The Negro to Black Conversion Experience" he explored how African Americans moved from being self-depreciating, self-hating "Negroes" to self-accepting, group appreciating "blacks" (Cross's article was written prior to the wide usage of the term "African American"). Cross's model offered a description of the coping strategies African Americans used to survive in a racist society. He argued that some of these coping mechanisms are psychologically healthy and self-promoting, while others are destructive and self-deprecating. In contrast to Cross's target-centered theory, the newer racial/cultural identity development models explain not only how minority group members view themselves, but also how racial/cultural minorities move from negative coping strategies to those that are more positive. In short, these models show how oppressed individuals develop a positive view of themselves and their race over time. As a result, racial/cultural identity development models have assisted counselors in understanding not only how minority clients view themselves fixed in time but also how the influence of oppression and racism impacts that view.

Since 1971, models of racial/cultural identity development have been designed for African Americans, (Vontress, 1971; Hall, Cross & Freedle, 1972; Jackson, 1975), Hispanics (Ruiz, 1990), women (Downing & Roush, 1985; McNamara & Rickard, 1989), gays and lesbians (Cass, 1979), people with disabilities (Olkin, 1999), and biracial/multiracial individuals (Poston, 1990). Most of these models were developed for specific ethnic or cultural groups. However, a couple of models are more inclusive and may address people of any ethnicity or culture (Atkinson, et al., 1979, 1989, 1998; Helms, 1995; Sue & Sue, 2003). For instance, Helms (1995) developed her People of Color model after much research on white and black models. Her model addresses the racial identities of all of the major racial minority groups in the United States—Asian, African, Latino and Latina, and Native American. Helms's model "is a derivative and integration of aspects of Cross's (1971) Negro-to-Black conversion model, Atkinson and colleagues' (1989) Minority Identity Development model, and Erikson's collective identity model, with some influence from Kohut's (1971) self psychology." (Helms & Cook, 1999, p. 86).

RACIAL/CULTURAL IDENTITY DEVELOPMENT OF OPPRESSED GROUPS

While there are strengths and weaknesses in all the models, the Sue and Sue (1990, 1999) model will be used for discussion here. This model was originally developed by Atkinson, Morten, and Sue (1979, 1989, 1998) and was named the Minority Development model. Sue and Sue later decided to develop a more inclusive model of identity development. Rather than focus on minority group members exclusively, the new Racial/Cultural Identity Development Model (R/CIDM), can be used across cultures and includes European Americans who are members of oppressed groups, such as women, gays, lesbians, bisexuals, trangendered individuals, and people with disabilities (Sue & Sue, 1990, 1999).

The R/CIDM may be used by minority counselors to determine their own identity development, and it is helpful in understanding how those who are different from them may perceive them. While the model does not predict client behaviors, it helps counselors understand those behaviors and avoid being shocked by them. Familiarity with the attitudes that accompany the stages can help counselors develop strategies for working effectively with individuals who have such attitudes.

The five stages of the R/CIDM are Conformity, Dissonance, Resistance, Introspection, and Integrative Awareness.

Conformity Stage

During the Conformity Stage, individuals carry a negative view of self, and they do not consider race to be an important factor in their lives. They disparage other oppressed groups as well as their own. In fact, individuals at this stage only appreciate the dominant white European American group.

For example, Maria, a Hispanic female made the following comment to her career counselor:

Joey told me that I was lucky because I was bilingual and could get a job anywhere. I hate that he just assumed that I speak Spanish because I am Hispanic. I asked him "Did you ever hear me speak Spanish? Do I speak with a Spanish accent?" I speak better English than most of them, and when I get work, I expect the people I work with to know how to speak English—I don't understand why people think they should get a job in this country without knowing how to speak English.

Dissonance Stage

Stage 2 is called the Dissonance Stage, because individuals at this stage have discovered that discrimination and oppression exist, and they are conflicted about it. They are still self-deprecating about their own race/culture, but they see some merit within their own group. Their new knowledge about oppression also makes them conflicted in their views of other oppressed groups. Individuals at this stage begin to question the dominant group—sometimes appreciating it and sometimes disapproving of it.

For example, a high school student in her school counselor's office stated the following:

I saw this program on TV last night about how people who have ethnic sounding names can't get jobs. I'm glad my parents gave me an American name, but if they named me Ashanti and I was qualified for the job, what difference should it make what my name is? Maybe it's because employers have to think about how their customers would react to someone's name if it is different. I still don't think it is fair.

Resistance Stage

At the Resistance Stage, people are joyous about their racial heritage. Their connection with other oppressed groups is primarily focused on joining with them to defeat the oppressor. They hold the dominant group, white European Americans, responsible for all of their own group's problems, and anything associated with the dominant group is rejected.

For example, an African American elementary school teacher said the following:

We have to get more African American counselors in the schools, because these white counselors are keeping black children in special education classes and ruining their chance to have a decent life. We need to get into the schools and take care of our own to stop this educational genocide.

Introspection Stage

Individuals at the Introspection Stage begin to doubt the extremity of the "we're all good, they are all bad" stance of the Resistance Stage. These individuals think that there are probably two sides to the issue of oppression. At this stage, individuals begin to pull away from the group position, and they are eager to learn about oppression from other oppressed groups, while choosing acceptable members of the dominant group to trust. Although they have begun to appreciate aspects of the dominant society, they still worry about selling out their own people (Sue & Sue, 2003, p. 222).

For example, a European American female medical student said the following to her counselor:

In my internship I'm assigned to a male OB-GYN, and he is the most gentle and caring doctor I have ever seen. The women's medical student group I belong to believes that only women can be good gynecologists, and so did I. It's why I wanted to enter this specialty to begin with—to give women better choices in their health care. I had never ever met an understanding male OB-GYN before. It's weird. I'm almost afraid to tell the other women about how good he is.

Integrative Awareness Stage

Finally, individuals achieve a positive racial/cultural identity when they reach the Integrative Awareness Stage. They appreciate themselves as racial/cultural beings, they appreciate their own group, and they appreciate other groups. They understand and empathize with the stages of racial identity development of others. As far as the dominant group is concerned, they have not reverted to the conformity stage in their appreciation, but instead they choose to trust individuals from the dominant group who are also engaged in combating oppression.

For instance, an Asian American supervisor said the following to a Japanese American employee:

Tamiko, I understand how angry you became when you discovered that you did not get the promotion. I understand how you could believe that it was a racist decision to promote a white woman over you when you have worked here longer. As an Asian woman, I did everything I could to insure that we exploited all of our resources when recruiting minorities for this position. I am certain that every minority applicant was thoroughly considered. I have outlined the reason why we chose the other woman, and I assure you that I confronted the committee on the issue of race throughout the hiring process. I feel confident that a fair decision has been made. I only hope that one day, Tamiko, you will understand our decision.

WHITE RACIAL IDENTITY DEVELOPMENT

While the racial/cultural identity models promote understanding oppression from the target's point of view, white racial identity models help us understand oppression from the perspective of privilege. Several models of white racial identity have been created (Carney & Kahn, 1984; Hardiman, 1982; Helms, 1984, 1990, 1994, 1995; Terry, 1977; Rowe et al., 1994). Each was developed to increase understanding of white dominance, racism, discrimination, and/or privilege. Hardiman (1982) conducted a qualitative study of white Americans and discovered that these individuals go through five stages of development before they reach a level of racial/cultural consciousness that is nonracist. The Rowe, Bennett, and Atkinson (1994) model is somewhat different from the Hardiman model in that it (a) does not propose a developmental stage model but describe types of racial consciousness between which individuals can move, and (b) it divides people into two categories—those whose positive racial identity has been "achieved" and those whose positive racial identity has been "unachieved." In another study, Ponterotto, Gretchen, and Utsey (2002) and Sabnani and colleagues (1991) concentrate on the racial/cultural identity development of counselors in training, and they provide training suggestions that will promote growth and development in their counseling students.

When the characteristics discussed in the Sue and Sue (2003) model, as outlined in the above section, are applied to white European Americans, these characteristics may be somewhat reversed. For example, during the Conformity Stage, acceptance of the dominant cultural group means acceptance of one's own group, which is the reverse of this same characteristic when applied to oppressed groups. However, some characteristics stay the same. Regardless of group membership, the cultures of oppressed groups are rejected in the conformity stage. Sue and Sue (2003) go on to describe how each of the stages can be applied to whites. (For a fuller description of this model, please refer to Sue & Sue, 2003.)

Instead of continuing with Sue and Sue's model to describe white racial identity, Helms's (1984) white racial identity model will be outlined here, as it is the most sophisticated, well known, widely researched (and perhaps most controversial) model of white racial identity to date. In contrast to the Sue and Sue R/CIDM model, Helms contends that because of the perception that stages are static and unchangeable, she decided to use the word "status" instead of "stages" in her identity development model. According to Helms, this was necessary to "encourage mental health workers who use racial identity models to conceive of the process of development as involving dynamic evolution rather than static personality structures or types," (Helms & Cook, 1999, p. 84). In other words, the word "status" reflects the process by which white individuals respond to race-based information. While the simplest status always develops first, white individuals have the potential to develop the other statuses as they mature. The status that receives the most reinforcement is likely to become dominant. Listed below are the white Racial Identity (WRI) status levels as devised by Helms.

Contact Status

The Contact Status is the one in which most whites begin their journey toward positive racial/cultural identity. During this status, individuals deny that race is important or that racism exists. They are unaware of race privilege, they accept current race relations as they are, and they avoid racial issues in general.

For example, a counselor in the Contact Status might say:

I believe in Person-Centered counseling, and if I am accepting and respectful of my clients, I don't see why I need to learn anything specific about their culture or about multicultural counseling. I've never had a client dislike me because I'm white.

Disintegration Status

The Disintegration Status occurs when white individuals have been confronted with the reality of oppression and they are forced to choose between former misinformed beliefs and morality. If they continue to support oppression through denial of its existence, they are condoning mistreatment of fellow human beings. However, they most likely will not know how to handle the situation effectively.

For example, a counselor in the Disintegration Status might say:

I'm very frustrated about the attrition rate of ethnic minority clients in our drop-out prevention program. Nothing we do seems to be working, but I don't have a clue what does work. Maybe we just need to hire more minority counselors who can do the job with clients more effectively.

Reintegration Status

In the Reintegration Status, white individuals retreat back to their own racial group and denigrate other racial groups. Individuals in this status have typically experienced such anxiety and pain while in the Disintegration Status that they seek relief via traditional justifications for oppression, thus relinquishing their own responsibility for it.

For example, a person in the Reintegration Status might say something blatantly racist and seek justification for it from another person, such as:

Look, I've tried to train some of those black workers, but they just don't get it. I don't know why they let people like that in this company anyway. You know Jack's cousin couldn't get a job here, but they hire all these blacks on Affirmative Action.

Pseudo-Independence (P-I) Status

Individuals at the P-I Status have developed an intellectual understanding of oppression and identify with nonoppressive whites. Helms & Cook (1999) describes this stage as an "intellectual commitment to one's own socioracial group." (p. 92) During P-I, whites are most accepting of those oppressed group members who are most like themselves, and they are committed to helping those who are dissimilar to themselves to learn how to assimilate.

For example, someone in the P-I Status might say:

I had a wonderful Latina student in my office this morning. She says that she wants to be a doctor and she has really good grades, so she could do it. The problem is that she has such a heavy accent, I'm not sure how well she will do at the university level. I'm going to see if I can get her into one of those speech classes that they have at the community college—you know the ones that help you speak Standard English and get rid of your accent. I'm sure she'll do great in it because she is so young.

Immersion Status

In the Immersion Status, white individuals attempt to redefine their whiteness. They search for the truth regarding oppression and immerse themselves in this topic.

For example, a white female law student in the Immersion Status might say:

I know that this university must be discriminating against ethnic minorities because there are so few here as compared to other law schools. I've gotten together with a couple of students to research the admissions criteria. It will help me to understand why I was accepted and why African American applicants, like my friend Julie, who is brilliant, was not.

Autonomy Status

Individuals at Autonomy Status level have reached the most advanced level of white racial identity. Not only have they accepted and embraced their own racial group, but they also understand and reject unearned privileges of race and avoid people who are racist and otherwise oppressive.

For example, someone in the Autonomy Status might say:

I had a client today who was really hurting. He says that he was let go from his job, but a younger, less experienced Asian American employee was retained. He is so bitter about all racial groups. It is going to be a challenge to work with him, but I think I saw a glimmer of hope when I asked him if there had ever been any people of color he liked and he said yes.

I'm going to need some support with this one because it has been a very long time since I have even been exposed to someone who was so racist.

DEVELOPING A POSITIVE RACIAL IDENTITY

Certainly, everyone who reads about racial identity development would like to believe that he or she has reached the highest level of development. However, most people who take a closer look at their attitudes and behaviors may find that their racial identity attitudes are not quite as developed as they would like. This is not a problem because there are a great many ideas and exercises to help in developing a positive racial identity (Arredondo et al., 1996; Helms, 1992; Parker, 1998; Sabnani, Ponterotto & Borodowsky, 1991). An excellent source for exploring white racial identity development is Helms's (1992), *A Race Is a Nice Thing to Have: A Guide to Being a White Person or Understanding the White Persons in Your Life*. You may also want to try some of the growth exercises below.

Activities for Developing a Positive Racial Identity

Conformity/Contact Stage/Status

Do research on oppression by reading diaries, autobiographies, and historical accounts written by members of your own racial/cultural group. For example, European Americans should read autobiographies and biographies of whites who both opposed and approved of slavery to have a greater understanding of the times and the evolution of slavery (e.g., William Lloyd Garrison, Lucretia Mott, Jefferson Davis).

Dissonance/Disintegration Stage/Status

Research the history of other racial/cultural groups. Read the literature of those groups as written by member of those groups, including both their popular publications (e.g., magazines) and novels. Take field trips to visit museums devoted to the lives of other cultural groups. Do some reading on white privilege and talk to others about how it affects you.

Resistance/Reintegration Stage/Status

Read research articles on racial/cultural identity development models. Pay special attention to those articles that discuss the emotional characteristics and effects of the various developmental stages/statuses. Read literature (novels, poetry, essays, autobiographies, biographies, etc.) on the effects of racism and oppression on all groups—not just the target group. When reading biographies/autobiographies of/by individuals involved in anti-oppression work, try to determine where those individuals would fall in the racial/cultural identity development model.

Pseudo-Independent Status (No Parallel under R/CIDM)

Write about your own experiences as a white person. Keep a journal of your feelings when you are in a racially/culturally mixed environment. Develop closer relationships with people of color so that you can honestly talk about your feelings about race and racial differences. Realize when you are comfortable and uncomfortable around people of color, but make efforts to leave your comfort zone so that you can add to your knowledge about others.

Immersion Status (No Parallel under R/CIDM)

Find a role model who has moved through the stage/status you are trying to get through. Join clubs and organizations of people who are devoted to making positive changes in racial/cultural relationships. Read about the journeys of others who have fought racism and oppression—especially those who are members of your own racial or cultural group.

Introspection Stage (No Parallel under WRI)

The confusion about whether or not all whites (men, heterosexuals, able-bodied, etc.) are bad may be remedied by getting more information. Reading biographies and histories about white abolitionists and civil rights workers, male feminists, and heterosexual friends of gays, lesbians, bisexual and transgender individuals would be very helpful at this stage. Locating such individuals who are active in winning rights for oppressed people and talking with them about their commitment to the causes of social justice may go a long way toward transcending this stage.

Autonomy/Internalization Stage/Status

Increase your exposure to a variety of racial and cultural groups. Research and become an active participant in organizations designed to promote social advocacy and anti-oppression.

FINAL THOUGHTS ABOUT CULTURE

Awareness of one's own race and culture is the first step towards multicultural competence. Too often, it is a step that is skipped or glossed over. It is a great deal more difficult to have an appreciation and respect for the cultures of others when one has no appreciation for one's own culture. Ottavi, Pope-Davis, and Dings (1994) in their research on white counseling students, found that students' racial/cultural identity was significantly related to their perceptions of their own multicultural counseling competence. They recommended, therefore, that racial/cultural identity development needs to be a significant part of training new counselors. Knowing the importance of your own cultural values and beliefs prepares you for the challenges you will face when you encounter clients with different cultural values and beliefs.

REVIEW/REFLECTION QUESTIONS

1. Given the readings and exercises you have completed in this chapter, how would you now describe your culture to someone? How does this definition compare to how you would have described your culture before reading this chapter?

2. Cultural value orientations (worldviews) are very important in the lifestyles of both client and counselor. What would be some of the challenges in working with career clients whose value orientations differ from the dominant culture regarding time, human activity, and relationship with the world?

3. Racial/cultural identity development is an essential concept for the culturally competent counselor to understand. How would you describe racial/cultural identity to someone who has never heard of the concept? What would you emphasize as the most important aspect of racial/cultural identity to career counselors?

REFERENCES

Arredondo, P., Toporek, R., Brown, S. P., Jones, J., Locke, D. C., Sanchez, J., & Stadler, H. (1996). Operationalization of the multicultural counseling competencies. *Journal of Multicultural Counseling and Development, 24*, 42–78.

Atkinson, D. R., Morten, G., & Sue, D. W. (1979). *Counseling American minorities: A cross-cultural perspective.* Dubuque, IA: Brown.

Atkinson, D. R., Morten, G., & Sue, D. W. (1989). A minority identity development model. In D. R. Atkinson, G. Morten & D. W. Sue (Eds.), *Counseling American Minorities* (pp. 35–52). Dubuque, IA: Brown.

Atkinson, D. R., Morten, G., & Sue, D. W. (1998). *Counseling American Minorities* (5th ed). Boston: McGraw-Hill.

Axelson, J. A. (1999). *Counseling and development in a multicultural society.* Pacific Grove, CA: Brooks/Cole Publishing Company.

Carney, C. G., & Kahn, K. B. (1984). Building competencies for effective cross-cultural counseling: A developmental view. *The Counseling Psychologist, 12,* 111–119.

Carter, R. T., Gushue, G. V., & Weitzman, L. M. (1994). White racial identity development and work values. *Journal of Vocational Behavior, 44,* 185–197.

Cass, V. C. (1979). Homosexual identity formation: A theoretical model. *Journal of Homosexuality, 4,* 219–235.

Cross, W. E. (1971). The Negro-to-Black conversion experience: Toward a psychology of Black liberation. *Black World, 20,* 13–27.

Downing, N. E., & Roush, K. L. (1985). From passive acceptance to active commitment: A model of feminist identity development for women. *Counseling Psychologist, 13,* 695–709.

Evans, K. M., & Herr, E. L. (1994). The influence of racial identity and the perception of discrimination on the career aspirations of African American men and women. *Journal of Vocational Behavior, 44,* 173–184.

Gollnick, D. M., & Chinn, P. C. (1994). *Multicultural education in a pluralistic society.* New York: Merrill.

Haley, A. (1990). *Exploring your heritage.* A presentation given at the College of William and Mary, Williamsburg, VA.

Hall, W. S., Cross, W. E., & Freedle, R. (1972). Stages in the development of Black awareness: An exploratory investigation. In R. L. Jones (Ed.). *Black Psychology* (pp. 156–165). New York: Harper & Row.

Hardiman, R. (1982). *White identity development: A process oriented model for describing the racial consciousness of White Americans.* Unpublished doctoral dissertation, University of Massachusetts, Amherst.

Helms, J. E. (1984). Toward a theoretical explanation of the effects of race on counseling: A Black and White model. *The Counseling Psychologist, 12,* 153–165.

Helms, J. E. (1990). *Black and White racial identity: Theory, research, and practice.* New York: Greenwood Press.

Helms, J. E. (1994). Racial identity and other "racial" constructs. In E. J. Trickett, R. Watts & D. Birman (Eds.), *Human Diversity* (pp. 285–311). San Francisco: Jossey Bass.

Helms, J. E. (1995). An update of Helms's White and people of color racial identity models. In J. G. Ponterotto, J. M. Casas, L. A. Suzuki & C. M. Alexander (Eds.). *Handbook of multicultural counseling* (pp. 181–191). Thousand Oaks, CA: Sage.

Helms, J. E. (1992). *A race is a nice thing to have: A guide to being a White person or understanding the White persons in your life.* Topeka, KS: Content Communications.

Helms, J. E., & Cook, D. A. (1999). *Using race and culture in counseling and psychotherapy: Theory and process.* Needham Heights, MA: Allyn & Bacon, 1999.

Helms, J. E., & Piper, R. E. (1994). Implicaitons of racial identity theory for vocational psychology. *Journal of Vocational Behavior, 44,* 124–138.

Hines, A., & Pedersen, P. (1980). The cultural grid: Matching social system variables and cultural perspectives. *Asian Pacific Training Development Journey, 1,* 5–11.

Ibrahim, F. A. (1991). Contribution of cultural worldview to generic counseling and development. *Journal of Counseling and Development, 70,* 13–19.

Ibrahim, F. A., & Kahn, H. (1984). *Scale to assess worldview (SAWV).* Unpublished document.

Ibrahim, F. A., & Kahn, H. (1987). Assessment of world views. *Psychological Reports, 60,* 163–176.

Jackson, B. (1975). Black identity development. *Journal of Educational Diversity, 2,* 19–25.

Kluckhohn, F. R., & Strodtbeck, F. L. (1961). *Variations in value orientations.* Evanston, IL: Row, Patterson, & Co.

Kohut, H. (1971). *Analysis of the self.* New York: International University Press.

Lee, C. (1995). School counseling and cultural diversity: A framework for effective practice. In C. C. Lee (Ed.). *Counseling for diversity: A guide for school counselors and related professionals* (pp. 3–17). Needham Heights, MA: Allyn & Bacon, 1995.

McGrath, P., & Axelson, J. A. (1999). *Accessing awareness and developing knowledge: Foundations for skill in a multicultural society.* Pacific Grove, CA: Brooks/Cole Publishing.

McNamara, K., & Rickard, K. M. (1989). Feminist identity development: Implications for feminist therapy with women. In D. R. Atkinson & G. Hackett (Eds.), *Counseling diverse populations* (2nd ed., pp. 271–282). Boston: McGraw-Hill.

Myers, H. F., Wohlford, P., Guzman, L. P., & Echemendia, R. J. (Eds.). (1991). *Ethnic minority perspectives on clinical training and services in psychology.* Washington, DC: American Psychological Association.

Olkin, R. (1999). *What psychotherapists should know about disability.* New York: Guilford.

Ottavi, T. M., Pope-Davis, D. B., & Dings, J. G. (1994). Relationship between white racial identity attitudes and self-reported multicultural counseling competencies. *Journal of Counseling Psychology, 41,* 149–154.

Parker, W. M. (1998). *Consciousness-raising: A primer for multicultural counseling* (2nd ed.). Springfield, IL: Charles C Thomas.

Pedersen, P. (1994). *A handbook for developing multicultural awareness* (2nd ed.). Alexandria, VA: American Counseling Association.

Pedersen, P. (Ed.). (1999). *Multiculturalism as a fourth force.* Philadelphia: Brunner/Mazel.

Ponterotto, J. G., Gretchen, D., & Utsey, S. O. (2002). A revision of the multicultural counseling awareness scale. *Journal of Multicultural Counseling & Development, 30*(3), 153–180.

Poston, W. S. (1990). The biracial identity development model: A needed addition. *Journal of Counseling and Development, 69,* 152–155.

Ridley, C. R., Liddle, M. C., & Li, L. C. (2001). Ethical decision-making in multicultural counseling. In J. G. Ponterotto, J. M. Casas, L. A. Suzuki & C. M. Alexander (Eds.) (pp. 165–188). *Handbook of multicultural counseling* (2nd ed.). Thousand Oaks, CA: Sage Publications.

Rowe, W., Bennett, S. K., & Atkinson, D. R. (1994). White racial identity models: A critique and alternative proposal. *The Counseling Psychologist, 22,* 129–146.

Ruiz, A. S. (1990). Ethnic identity: Crisis and resolution. *Journal of Multicultural Counseling and Development, 18,* 29–40.

Sabnani, H. B., Ponterotto, J. G., & Borodowsky, L. G. (1991). White racial identity development and cross-cultural counselor training: A sage model. *The Counseling Psychologist, 19,* 76–102.

Sire, J. (1976). *The Universe Next Door: A Basic World-View.* InterVarsity Press.

Sue, D. W. (1978). Worldviews and counseling. *Personnel and Guidance Journal, 56,* 458–462.

Sue, D. W., & Sue, D. (1990). *Counseling the culturally different: Theory and practice.* New York: Wiley.

Sue, D. W., & Sue, D. (1999). *Counseling the culturally different: Theory and practice* (3rd ed.). New York: Wiley.

Sue, D. W., & Sue, D. (2003). *Counseling the culturally different.* New York: John Wiley & Sons, Inc.

Swim, J. K., Cohen, L. L., & Hyers, L. L. (1998). Experiencing everyday prejudice and discrimination. In J. K. Swim & C. Stangor (Eds.) *Prejudice: The target's perspective* (pp. 37–60). San Diego, CA: Academic Press.

Terry, R. W. (1977). *For whites only.* Grand Rapids, MI: William B. Erdmans.

Trevino, J. G. (1996). Worldview and change in cross-cultural counseling. *The Counseling Psychologist, 24,* 198–215.

Vontress, C. E. (1971). Racial differences: Impediments to rapport. *Journal of Counseling Psychology, 18,* 7–13.

CHAPTER 3
Your Biases

In order to become a culturally competent career counselor, it is important not only to understand one's own culture, as discussed in the previous chapter, but also to understand one's culture as it relates to working with people from other cultures. When counselors believe that their own cultural perspective is the only way to see and deal with the world, there is a problem. Wrenn (1962) described this phenomenon as cultural encapsulation. Cultural encapsulation is a symptom of racism and prejudice; it perpetuates oppression, because the belief in the superiority of one's own culture would mean that other cultures are inferior and deserve to be treated as such. One would hope that today the number of culturally encapsulated counselors is small. The challenge, therefore, is not simply to increase counselor awareness of the dangers of cultural encapsulation but more specifically to help them identify and eliminate cultural encapsulation in their practice.

The discussion of prejudices and biases involves some historical reflection. A review of U.S. history is not intended here. Instead, the focus is to encourage potential career counselors to review their personal histories of prejudice, racism, and bias.

At the beginning stages of life, people have no biases and prejudices. During infancy, children have an endless curiosity, and rather than approaching strange people or things with the assumption that they are good or bad, they are just curious about them. Gradually, children learn about "others" (those who are different from them and their families). They also begin to understand how the significant people in their lives feel about the others and how others are treated by society and the media. Through these latter experiences biases and prejudices begin. Although no one is born having biases or prejudices, everyone learns them. Children are typically praised, accepted, or encouraged when their opinions match those of significant adults. This reinforcement comes not only from the significant adults in their lives (parents, guardians, family members, teachers, neighbors), but also from the books they read, the television programs and movies they watch, and the impressions they gather watching interactions among strangers. When these factors contain negative connotations about "others," prejudices are born. The good news is that if biases and prejudices can be learned, they can also be unlearned. It is unlikely, however, that in changing their beliefs people will receive even a fraction of the positive reinforcement they earned when they learned to be prejudiced. It is more likely that they will be rejected or ridiculed by prejudiced peers for reducing their prejudices (D'Andrea and Daniels, 2001).

Because people learn biases and prejudices over their entire lifetimes, these prejudices are deeply embedded in their belief systems. Unlearning these biases is difficult and sometimes painful. This chapter may challenge readers' beliefs, and it may even hurt their feelings. I encourage readers to try to keep an open mind no matter which emotions may surface as they read. I urge readers to assume that at least part of what they read about their prejudices and biases may be true. It is only in doing this kind of self-reflection that readers will be able to conquer their biases and prejudices and develop into culturally competent career counselors. Four manifestations of bias will be discussed in detail: stereotyping, prejudice, racism and oppression, and privilege.

STEREOTYPING

An innate cognitive process that is common to all humans is the propensity to categorize things and people into groups. This tendency for classification, though, is useful in certain situations, such as scientific categorization of the natural world and organizing one's home or office. However, this innate propensity can also lead to stereotyping, which is the root of biased beliefs and behaviors. Everyone learns to stereotype to simplify complicated information, and so, unfortunately, the complexity of U.S. populations is ripe for stereotyping. If a few people in a group share certain traits, it is easier for people to simplify matters by generalizing the similar characteristics of those few persons to all members of the group rather than understanding the differences among the group members. In conjunction with making stereotypical generalizations themselves, people may also learn about group stereotypes from others, which only reinforces their own generalizations. While stereotypical categorization is problematic in itself, the more compelling problem is that most stereotypes carry negative connotations, thus laying a foundation for prejudice. "A stereotype and a prejudice are similar only in that they both contain elements that are false or inaccurate, invoke emotional feeling, and result from routinized habits of judgment and expectations" (Axelson, 1999, pg. 49). Axelson has outlined some of the common characteristics of stereotypes.

- They are *pervasive* in that most people have their own "pet" personality theories about the characteristics of others.
- They tend to emphasize *differences* when applied to individuals or groups different from oneself but to emphasize *similarities* when applied to individuals or groups similar to oneself.
- They tend to be *biased* more by socioeconomic status roles than by ethnicity when applied to characteristics of individuals and groups different from oneself or one's own group; and they tend to be *negative* if the stereotype serves as transmission for prejudice.
- They tend to become *habitual* and *routinized* unless challenged.
- *First impressions* are usually based on stereotypes.
- *New stereotypes* will supplement or supplant existent stereotypes as conditions and experiences in the culture change.
- Stereotyping and stereotypes *impair* the ability to assess others accurately and can readily lead to misinterpretations (p. 50).

The following exercises are designed to help readers to assess the extent to which they stereotype individuals and groups and to help them break these habits.

Overcoming Stereotyping Exercise

It is extremely difficult to admit to stereotyping. Most people who hold stereotypical views have normalized their views as a perfectly natural response to complex data. To break free from this normalized perspective, try to view stereotypes in a different manner.

In this exercise, you are asked to use your own personal and cultural standards regarding work as an avenue for exploring your stereotypes toward others. In the spaces below, write down:

(a) Your perception of success. How does a person become successful? How does a person know when he or she is successful?

_____

_____

_____

(b) Your work ethic. What makes a good worker? What is important about the work one does?

_____

_____

_____

(c) What personality characteristics are important for workers to possess?

_____

_____

_____

After you have completed writing about your standards for work, write another paragraph expressing your thoughts about yourself and how well you live up to the standards you have just written. What are your thoughts about family members who do not meet these standards?

_____

_____

_____

_____

_____

Once you have taken a good look at your own standards, think about what you have heard about the standards of other groups (their standards of success, their work ethic, their personality characteristics) and how those attributes measure up to your standards. Knowing that no one, including you, is likely to meet all of your standards will give you permission to question stereotypes.

Career Stereotypes Exercise

This exercise focuses on imagery.

List below five high-status careers, five medium-level careers, and five low-status careers (you define which careers fit which categories). As you are listing each career, write down the first image that comes to mind regarding the person representing each career. What does that person look like? What is that person's race or ethnicity, sexual orientation, gender, ability status? (For example, what image comes to mind when you think of: college professors, funeral directors, housekeepers, designers, nurses?) Next, write down someone in that same career who is completely different from your original image. Keep going with the imagery until you have covered all three lists.

High-status careers

1. _____

_____

2. _____

_____

3. _____

_____

4. _____

_____

5. _____

_____

Medium-level careers

1. _____

_____

2. _____

_____

3. _____

_____

4. _____

_____

5. _____

_____

Low-status careers

1. _____

_____

2. _____

_____

3. _____

_____

4. _____

_____

5. _____

_____

What did you think and feel during the imagery exercises? What did you learn about your career stereotypes? Perhaps, you found that some stereotypes were harder to imagine than others because some fields have become more diverse over time. The easier it is to imagine one type of person in a career, the stronger the stereotype.

Exploring Non-traditional Career Paths Exercise

Exploring stereotypes may involve examining the history of specific groups and identifying the jobs that were open to members of that group given the political and economic climate in the country at the time. For this exercise, do research on individuals who have entered career areas that are non-stereotypical for their specific groups (such as African American scientists, Asian American clinical psychologists, gay police officers, female engineers, and so forth). Discovering the stories of these individuals and the obstacles they had to overcome will help you to understand how entrenched stereotypes can be. Write down a brief summary of your research below:

_____

_____

_____

_____

_____

Label Exercise

A great collaborative classroom exercise for combating stereotypes is an adaptation of Pedersen's (1994) "Label Awareness Exercise" (p. 73). Pre-print one- or two-word stereotypes that have historically been applied to various oppressed groups on 8.5 × 11 paper. The labels can represent personality traits, job titles, or stereotypically insulting phrases, such as "lazy," "laundry owner," "on welfare," "good dancer," "stingy," "inscrutable," "drunk," "bitchy," and so forth. Then attach each label to the back of each student in the class so that the wearers cannot see the labels they are wearing. The students will then walk around the class for about ten minutes treating their classmates according to their labels. The label wearers must guess, based on how they are treated, what stereotypical labels they are wearing. Students find this a fun activity, they learn a lot about the power of labels, and they learn to empathize with individuals who are often assigned these labels in real life.

Stereotype Hunt Exercise

To reduce your tendency to stereotype, start practicing visualizing diverse people in the careers you routinely encounter, and notice when a stereotype causes you to do a double-take. For example, such a double-take occurred in the following scenario:

I recall flying from New York to Florida a few years ago, and once the plane was at cruising altitude, a female voice came over the intercom, and I immediately stopped listening, thinking that it was probably the flight attendant informing us about the beverage service. When the voice went on for a while talking about the altitude and winds, I realized that it was the pilot speaking. I was really embarrassed because two of my occupational stereotypes had been challenged—all flight attendants are women and all pilots are men.

Career counselors should learn to understand stereotyping and its characteristics by researching work stereotypes of various oppressed groups. This research will reveal the origins of the stereotypes and help counselors to separate fact from fiction. Associating clients with careers because of race, ethnicity, gender, sexual orientation, or ability status is the first step to avoid in multicultural career counseling. Because prejudice starts with stereotyping, an understanding of origins and harmful effects of stereotypes will help career counselors to begin to reduce their prejudices.

PREJUDICE

So much about prejudice and racism is intertwined that most people use the terms interchangeably. However, the terms are not one and the same. Allport (1979) defined prejudice as "thinking ill of others without sufficient warrant; or incorporating a bipolar (negative and positive) component as in 'a feeling,' favorable or unfavorable, toward a person or thing, prior to or based on actual experience" (p. 6). Just as the word implies, prejudice involves making a judgment before having the facts—a pre-judgment. Ridley (1995) defines racism as "any behavior or pattern of behavior that tends to systematically deny access to opportunities or privileges to members of one racial group while perpetuating access to opportunities and privileges to members of another racial group" (p. 28). To expand Ridley's definition slightly, note that it may also be applied to groups oppressed in other ways not based on race, such as white women, persons with disabilities, gay/lesbian/bisexual/transgendered persons, and so forth. Thus Ridley's definition is also a definition of oppression in general. While prejudice is typically attitudinal, oppression involves behavior. Oppression "always involves harmful behavior, whereas . . . prejudice involves only negative attitudes, beliefs, and intentions. Herein lies the major differences between these two phenomena. [Oppression] is behavioral and prejudice is dispositional" (Ridley, 1995, p. 18).

According to Dovidio, Kawakami, and Gaetner (2000), prejudice can also entail a passive behavioral component. In their view, prejudice consists of three components: cognitive, affective, and behavioral. For example, an individual may think that poor people are too lazy to work hard (cognitive component); or an individual may feel discomfort when having to socialize with gays and lesbians (affective component); or an individual may seek out and move to a segregated part of town, one in which only members of that person's own race, sexual orientation, ethnicity, and so forth live (behavioral component). In the last instance, the behavior becomes racist if the individual in the segregated neighborhood works to keep "others" out or condones such behavior.

Some may insist that they have been brought up to believe that everyone is equal, so therefore they have no prejudices. Having this kind of upbringing, however, does *not* insulate one from developing prejudices, especially if the lessons that were taught were purely cognitive. Prejudice can be passed from one generation to another without explicit lessons in prejudice. The old adage, "actions speak louder than words" is especially relevant when teaching about prejudice. For example, if an individual's parents or guardians always told a child that "people are people and we always respect people no matter what color or religion they are," but they nonetheless sent the child to segregated schools, lived in a segregated neighborhood, lacked friends from different cultural groups, never talked about race, or failed to react to racist behaviors of others, they have nevertheless communicated prejudice throughout the child's development (Ponterotto & Pedersen, 1993).

Likewise, even if a person's family and significant adults were vigilant about teaching acceptance of cultural differences through their words and deeds, education in prejudicial attitudes is still possible through mass communication. More so than one might want to believe, the media (newspapers, magazines, television) constantly promote prejudicial attitudes and perpetuate negative stereotypes of ethnic minorities and other oppressed groups (Ponterotto & Pedersen, 1993). For example, oppressed group members consistently play stereotypic work roles on many television shows (such as African American drug pushers, Latina maids and housekeepers, Asian restaurant owners, gay hair dressers and designers). The few ethnic minorities who portray doctors, lawyers, police officers, and other high-level professionals on television are often seen as having sold out to the white culture because in these programs they are rarely shown in the context of their own culture. Even more distressing is the absence of people with disabilities in career roles on television. Not to single out television, the print media also do little to promote positive career images of oppressed groups. It is not likely that members of oppressed groups are sought after as experts for newspapers and magazines unless there is a special topic devoted to the particular group the expert belongs to. Instead, ethnic minorities are more prominent in daily papers for committing crimes than they are for any socially acceptable careers they may engage in. These negative representations reinforce prejudicial attitudes toward members of minority groups by the entire society. Speaking metaphorically, avoiding prejudice is like avoiding air pollution. Even if people and their families drive ecologically friendly automobiles, they will still breathe in the pollution from cars that are not ecologically friendly.

Despite all evidence to the contrary, there is, sadly, an increasing number of people who truly believe that they are not prejudiced, even while they hold prejudicial attitudes toward oppressed groups. This phenomenon has been labeled "aversive racism" (Dovidio et al., 2000, p. 137). "Many people who consciously and sincerely support egalitarian principles and believe themselves to be non-prejudiced also unconsciously harbor negative feelings and beliefs about blacks (as well as about other historically disadvantaged groups)" (p. 138). Aversive racists, however, while not overtly anti-black or hostile to other racial and minority groups, are prejudiced insofar as they hold more positive beliefs about whites than they hold negative beliefs about blacks (Dovidio et al., 2000). For example, a white high school counselor cannot understand why his academically brilliant African American student chooses to attend a historically black college when she was accepted at one of the most prestigious white schools in the country. To this counselor, attending the white school would have been far better for this student's career aspirations than any of the historically black colleges and universities in the country. He does not believe that black schools are bad but that the white schools are better. This belief system will be explained further in the section on racism and oppression.

Career counselors who want to be culturally competent must start by exploring their own prejudices. This historical self-review will help counselors to restructure the cognitive component of their prejudices against oppressed groups. An understanding of affective and behavioral components of prejudice might be achieved by reducing or eliminating oppression and privilege, two further manifestations of bias that will be discussed below. In addition, exercises in that section will cover racism and oppression.

RACISM AND OPPRESSION

When used in conversation in a culturally diverse group, the words "racism" and "oppression" are emotionally charged words that often have the effect of shutting down conversation. The word "racism" in particular brings up images of angry mobs burning crosses, lynching, shouting obscenities, and spewing hate. Another likely image is that of an ignorant, tobacco-spitting bigot, the historical stereotype of a racist. The word "oppression," though more general, conjures similar images of oppression against a variety of groups, including the images of a husband who hands the crying baby to his wife, a drunken band of gay bashers, and the immaculately dressed upper-class person who places a handkerchief over his or her nose when encountering a homeless person.

Viewing the words "racism" and "oppression" in such starkly and stereotypically visual terms is a limited view that is detrimental for counselors who wish to become culturally competent. The belief that racism and oppression are matters of the historical past or the belief that the stereotypical confederate-flag-waving image of a racist oppressor could hardly apply to anyone with sophistication and education such as a counselor is simply erroneous. Until counselors are able to accept that they too can be racists and oppressors, they will not be able to work effectively across cultures. There are probably as many definitions of racism and oppression as there are authors who write about them. In fact, the meanings have become so complex that the term "racism" has been broken down into several subcategories such as cultural racism, institutional racism, collective racism, individual racism, and internalized racism. Some understanding of each of these terms is necessary, and note that the terms, while created to define types of racism, can also be expanded to apply to oppression in general.

- Institutional racism occurs when the structure of society or an organization permits the creation and sanctioning of laws, policies, and customs that perpetuate the superior status of one group while denying or limiting access to goods, status, and economic opportunity to other groups (Axelson, 1993; Helms & Cook, 1999; Jones, 1972; Kovel, 1970; Sue & Sue, 2003).

Institutional racism is responsible for discrimination in the workplace, and unfair practices within educational institutions and government. For example, if an agency sends out important notices to clients or customers printed only in English when the agency is located in an area with a large Spanish-speaking population, that is institutional racism.

- Collective racism is an informal type of institutional racism in that the policies are not written down but there is a collective response by members of one cultural group to deny access to opportunities of another cultural group (Utsey, Bolden & Brown, p. 318).

For example, even though in 1996, the Texaco oil company policy of nondiscrimination was clearly published and even though Texaco was engaged in multicultural education of its employees, Texaco executives were caught on audiotape making racist remarks about African American and Jewish people. The tapes lent support to a discrimination lawsuit levied by African American executives of the company. This is an example of collective racism because company practices of denying opportunities to specific groups existed, even if the company's written policy stated otherwise.

- Cultural racism has been defined by a number of authors (Utsey, Bolden, & Brown, 2001; Jones, 1972; Helms & Cook, 1999). In essence, cultural racism occurs when members of one cultural group believe in the superiority of their group and devalue the cultural practices, accomplishments, and creativity of other cultural groups.

For example, after President Bush's 2005 presidential address wishing everyone who celebrated it a happy Kwanzaa (a cultural celebration of African heritage by African Americans), a flood of reactions criticizing the celebration and its founder poured into news organizations, many stating that it was anti-Christian. Such reactions may be considered cultural racism in that one group belittles the practices and creativity of another cultural group.

- Internalized racism occurs when an individual internalizes the stereotypes and attitudes held by those who discriminate against his or her group (Axelson, 1993; Helms & Cook, 1999). According to Jones, internalized racism ". . . is defined as acceptance of negative messages by members of stigmatized races about their own abilities and intrinsic worth. It is characterized by their not believing in others who look like them and not believing in themselves. It involves accepting limitations to one's full humanity, including one's spectrum of dreams, one's right to self-determination, and one's range of allowable self-expression." It can be seen in an embracing of "Whiteness" (Jones, 2000), such as the use of hair straightening and bleaching creams by African Americans; self-devaluating oneself, such as when one rejects one's ancestral culture; and resigning oneself to feelings of resignation, helplessness, and hopelessness, such as dropping out of school and engaging in risky health practices (Jones, 2000).
- Individual racism refers to the discriminatory behaviors of a single individual. These behaviors are based on racial prejudice and a belief in the individual's own genetic superiority (Axelson, 1999; Ponterotto & Pedersen, 1993). While institutional, cultural, and collective racism are of great concern in career counseling because they affect the career futures of clients, individual racism receives the greatest attention in career counseling literature and in training. The multicultural competencies require counselors to understand and overcome their own individual racism.

Some definitions of racism or oppression suggest that behavior is not racist or oppressive unless the perpetrator has power and or is supported by a powerful institution. In this definition, if a person does not have the power to do harm to another person, that person may hold prejudicial attitudes but is not considered racist or oppressive. Therefore, minority group members are typically not considered guilty of racism or oppression against the dominant group. The position taken in this text is that this distinction is moot when applied to the ethical behavior of counselors. Whether or not counselors work for institutions that condone prejudicial attitudes and racist or oppressive behavior, and whether or not they belong to the dominant or minority group, if the result of counselor behavior toward a client is harmful, the counselor is considered to have behaved unethically. For instance, if a gay Latino career counselor intentionally or unintentionally supplies fewer referrals to his heterosexual male clients than to his gay clients, the counselor's actions will be considered unethical.

Charles Ridley is perhaps the most cited author in regard to the relationship between racism (and by extension, other forms of group oppression) and counseling. It goes without saying that most counselors want to help, and it can be argued that very few counselors are likely to participate in overt and intentional racist or oppressive behaviors. However, Ridley's (1989; 1995) work has helped counselors to understand that even though they may not intend to hurt their clients, they can be guilty of racist behavior. Ridley (1995) contends that "[i]ntentions should not be used as the criteria for determining whether or not a behavior is racist . . . racial prejudice does not always cause racism. . . . A useful rule for determine racism is to look at behavior consequences first and motivation second. Regardless of a counselor's motivation, actual clinical behavior is what affects a client" (pp. 20–21). In other words, if the end result of a behavior is that specific groups of clients are systematically denied access to opportunities, that behavior is racist. For example, consider the following scenario:

Joan is a white, female career counselor in a high school. She is devoted to all of her students and believes that she does not harbor prejudices and biases. Joan is responsible for matching students with professionals they can shadow for one day to learn about the life in the real world workplace. She is committed to matching minority students with professionals from their own backgrounds who can be role models for them. Two of her minority students are interested in careers for which Joan has only located white professionals as volunteer mentors. Joan is afraid that if she makes a cross-racial match, the students will get the idea that minority group members are not welcome in that profession. She decides to match the students with volunteer mentors from their own racial groups who work in relatively closely related fields, not with the white volunteer mentors employed in the exact fields the students desire to enter.

Joan's plan in the above scenario would lead minority students to miss a learning opportunity they might not have missed if they were white. Because Joan's behavior could be seen as resulting in harm to her minority clients, the behavior would be classified as racist or oppressive no matter how well intentioned it was.

Although traditional forms of overt prejudice and racism or oppression (depicted so graphically every week by the 1970s television character, Archie Bunker) have dramatically declined (Devine, Plant & Buswell, 2000) over the years, some trends in U.S. society are disturbing.

The first is an insidious form of racism identified earlier in this chapter as aversive racism. In this type of racism, core U.S. values like equality have been reinterpreted in such a way that the term "equality" becomes a weapon against the very group it was intended to help. For example, the word "equality" has been used to criticize Affirmative Action and other remedies for discrimination created to overcome hundreds of years of oppression. D'Andrea and Daniels (2001), and Dovidio and colleagues (2000) agree that this new form of racism or oppression may be caused by a fear of the loss of privileges amongst dominant groups (such as whites, men, heterosexuals, people without disabilities). Unfortunately, these attitudes have become more acceptable over time and, as a result, race privilege and privileges based on gender, sexual orientation, and so forth have been condoned under a reinterpreted definition of equality.

A second insidious form of racism has been labeled "color blind racial attitudes" (CoBRA) (Neville et al., 2001, p. 270). According to Neville and colleagues, CoBRA are different from individual racism because they lack the element of an assumption of superiority. Neville and colleagues list several attributes of CoBRA:

1. CoBRA are "new forms of racial attitude expressions that are separate from, but related to racial prejudice . . . characterized by (a) persistent negative stereotyping, (b) tendency to blame minorities . . . for racial disparities . . . and (c) resistance to ameliorate problematic social conditions" (p. 270).
2. CoBRA are ". . . cognitive schema suggesting race is unimportant coupled with feelings of anxiety about race" (p. 272).
3. CoBRA are multidimentional and "reflect multiple beliefs" in which individuals deny color or power differences (p. 273).

In short, CoBRA are ways of ignoring race while simultaneously allowing racial inequities to exist. A typical CoBRA attitude would be to fault the poor (who just happen to be mostly single African American women and Latinas) for having a number of children and living off welfare while denouncing a tax increase to cover the expense of adequate and affordable day care through local governmental revenue since it favors the poor over other types of families. Neville and colleagues point out that though the intent of CoBRA are to treat everyone equitably by a denial of differences, often the results will show inequities in counseling outcomes. In other words, ignoring differences does not make them disappear. When counselors acknowledge and celebrate the differences between themselves and their clients, clients benefit from the relationship.

In the multicultural counseling literature, racism/oppression is a topic that has been well researched and discussed. Because white male heterosexuals have long been in a position of privilege in U.S. society, and because white male heterosexuals have been socialized and rewarded for oppressive behavior, most of the research attention has been given to overcoming oppressive behaviors in this population. White counselors need to accept responsibility for their own racism and to deal with it in a non-defensive, guilt free manner" (Sue & Sue, 2003, p. 454). Using Ridley's definition of racism (and by extension, oppression), however, counselors who are members of oppressed groups also must understand how their prejudices against their own and other groups can result in racist or oppressive behavior. They also should be vigilant in monitoring how they use the power of the counseling relationship. If they harbor biases against their own or other groups along with the power of the counseling relationship, their work with these clients may be harmful and, therefore, racist or oppressive. The first step toward understanding one's own biases and prejudices is to understand how privilege affects behavior and beliefs, which will be discussed in the next section of this chapter. But before readers move on to the next topic, they should complete the following exercises (some designed for individuals and some collaborative) for overcoming prejudice and racism/oppression.

Personal Reflection Exercise

Almost everyone has experienced being treated unfairly. Getting in touch with the feelings that accompany unfair treatment is a helpful way to understand racism or oppression and prejudice. Identify in the spaces below an incident in which you were treated unfairly. Once you have identified the incident, write down all of the particulars about it—especially your thoughts and feelings. Writing down your observations about this event will concretize the experience, and your notes will be a resource for you as your multicultural training continues. This exercise is designed to help you empathize with oppressed groups, whether you are a member of an oppressed group or not. If you empathize with members of one group, it is difficult to mistreat members of other groups.

_____

_____

_____

_____

_____

Cultural Exposure Exercise

Start increasing your exposure to a culturally different group you may have prejudices about. Begin with low risk–minimal contact activities (Parker, 1998) if you are at all timid about facing your own prejudices or racism OR oppression. These low-risk activities do not require any person-to-person contact with a member of an oppressed group. Write down your impressions in the spaces below:

1. Read more about racism/oppression and prejudice from counseling texts (e.g. Ponterroto & Pedersen, 1993; Ridley, 1995).

_____

_____

_____

_____

_____

2. Do some research on discrimination lawsuits and affirmative action over the last ten years.

_____

_____

_____

_____

_____

3. Read biographies and autobiographies about those involved in the anti-racism struggle, the feminist movement, the gay rights movement, and the fight for people with disabilities.

_____

_____

_____

_____

_____

Personal Assessment Exercise

This exercise involves an assessment of your own prejudices and oppressive behaviors. It is much more likely that a person interested in counseling will need to combat aversive racism and CoBRA rather than overt, intentional racism, so assessing your own aversive racism and CoBRA is the focus here. Indicate below if you have ever thought about or used any of the following statements or statements closely related to them. Then write down why these statements might be considered evidence of bias (adapted from Ochs & Evans, 1993).

1. I don't see you as (black, white, Asian, Latino or Latina, Indian, gay, lesbian, disabled, and so forth), I see you as a person.

_____

_____

2. I don't know what's the matter with (insert oppressed group) after all other people suffer oppression too.

_____

_____

3. Well _____ are racists too.

_____

_____

4. I really don't know what to say when I'm around _____.

_____

_____

5. Some of my best friends are _____.

_____

_____

6. I'm afraid that I might be mugged, robbed, or terrorized by one of them.

_____

_____

7. I really cannot do anything about (racism, discrimination, oppression). It is not my problem. I have enough to worry about.

_____

_____

8. I don't have any prejudices against _____; I've never even met any of them.

_____

_____

9. I just feel overwhelmed with how much I have to learn about other cultures.

_____

_____

10. My brother/aunt /cousin/friend/neighbor, etc. didn't get a job because of Affirmative Action.

_____

_____

11. I don't see why we have to put everything we write into two languages. Non-English speakers are going to have to learn to speak English anyway if they want to succeed in this country.

_____

_____

12. I'd really prefer to buy a house in a less integrated area. Not that I object to living in a neighborhood with people of color, I'm just afraid the property values may decrease in the future.

_____

_____

If you have identified with even one of these statements, and you don't understand why that statement may be considered racist, then you have work to do on your racial attitudes.

Immersion Exercise

The most obvious strategy to work on racial issues is to spend more time with diverse populations. Your interaction should be not only with people of your own socioeconomic status level but also be with those whose incomes are lower and higher than your own. Also, if you simply spend more time with one person who is Japanese American, for example, you learn some information about that person, but if you spend time with a number of Asian Americans you will be able to identify the inter-group differences in language, religion, and traditions among Asian Americans. Once you have completed this exercise, write down your experience/impressions in the spaces below.

_____

_____

_____

_____

_____

_____

Cultural Guide Exercise

Get to know someone from a particular culture with whom you can get along and attend cultural events, ask questions, and employ your childlike curiosity in order to learn more (Arredondo et al., 1996; D'Andrea & Daniels, 2001; Dovidio et al., 2000). Write down your experience/impressions in the spaces below.

_____

_____

_____

_____

_____

_____

Visual Exercise

Watch films that address prejudice and racism or oppression, such as *Crash, Smoke Signals, Monster's Ball, Do the Right Thing, Mi Familia, Mona Lisa Smile,* and documentaries such as *Color of Fear* and *Brown Eyes, Blue Eyes, The Celluloid Closet.* Such films stimulate an emotional awareness of oppression that is more poignant than reading alone (Arredondo et al., 1996). In fact, it is best to view those films with others and to debrief afterwards because they are so powerful. Record your impression in the spaces below.

_____

_____

_____

_____

_____

_____

PRIVILEGE

A natural consequence of racism or oppression is that some people will be the beneficiaries of privileges while others are denied privilege. In the United States, white European Americans are the privileged group. However, most white people do not think of their "whiteness" as a privilege (Vera, Feagin & Gordon, 1995)—especially those who have suffered discrimination based on their gender, religion, sexual orientation, physical ability status, or socioeconomic status. A general definition of privilege is that it is an advantage based solely on an accident of birth. For most people, that definition brings to mind the most privileged in our society—a white, wealthy, heterosexual, able-bodied, Protestant, male. Most people born to an advantageous station in life do not consider themselves to be privileged. They believe that because they are hard-working individuals, they have legitimately earned all that they possess and that they deserve.

Often, privilege is invisible to those who are on the receiving end, who simply believe that their privileged lifestyle is the way life should be. Jackson (1999) compares privilege to gaining permanent admission to an exclusive club the day one is born. In Jackson's analogy, membership to this club is neither desired nor requested, and it is almost impossible to resign. Privilege exists whether or not we condone it or seek it out. The invisibility of white privilege to so many people is understandable, because in the United States, citizens are socialized from childhood to believe that their achievements will be valued by others and that they will be rewarded for their efforts. In other words, most people believe that all achievements are based on merit and fairness. If this were true, then it would be reasonable to assume that there is no such thing as race-based, gender-based, sexual orientation–based, and other forms of privilege (Crowfoot & Chesler, 1996; Haney & Hurtado, 1994; McIntosh, 1988). In America, privileges are so ingrained in the fabric of the nation that they are apparent only to those who are not so privileged. In her article "White privilege and male privilege: A personal account of coming to see correspondence through work in women's studies," Peggy McIntosh (1988) couldn't understand how men in our society seemed oblivious to their privileges when it was so obvious to her. As a way to explore the privileges she didn't have, she decided to explore those unearned privileges she did have as a white person. In her landmark paper, McIntosh (1988) created a list of some of these privileges, which are listed below:

- I can turn on the television or open to the front page of the paper and see people of my race widely represented.
- When I am told about our national heritage or about "civilization," I am shown that people of my color made it what it is.
- I can arrange to protect my children most of the time from people who might not like them.
- I can speak in public to a powerful male group without putting my race on trial.
- I am never asked to speak for all the people of my race.
- I can remain oblivious of the language and customs of persons of color who constitute the world's majority without feeling in my culture any penalty for such oblivion.

- If a traffic cop pulls me over or if the IRS audits my tax return, I can be sure I haven't been singled out because of my race.
- I can take a job with an affirmative action employer without having coworkers on the job suspect that I got it because of race (McIntosh, 1988).

As the author of the book you are holding, I have found that it helps people to explore their own privileges if I describe the ways that I, an African American woman, am privileged. A few examples are:

- I am able-bodied and can easily climb the stairs to my office building without thinking about cut-out sidewalks, disabled parking, or ramps into the building.
- I am comfortably middle class and I can easily purchase most of the items that are advertised on television if I want to buy them. I can fill my refrigerator with food and I can buy the clothes I need to keep warm.
- I am heterosexual, so I may legally marry someone in any state of the union. I can also openly display affection toward my partner without fear of disapproval or reprisal.
- I am a Protestant so not only can I openly practice my religion but I also know my office will be closed for me to observe my religious holidays.

Then to underscore the presence of white privilege, I describe ways that I (a highly educated person) lack privilege in U.S. society due to my color. They include:

- Though I can afford most items in my local grocery and drug stores, I cannot find stockings in my skin tone in those stores.
- I can rarely find a variety of greeting cards to send family and friends with people who look like me on the front.
- When my performance is criticized, I often question whether the criticism was because of what I did or because of my race or gender.
- When I buy a house, I have to be careful that my realtor understands what I mean when I say I want to live in a comfortably integrated community, one in which my racial and cultural heritage will be accepted and in which the neighbors who are not like me are not in a flight or fight mode.

Understanding privilege and its consequences is extremely important for the culturally competent career counselor. To understand privilege is to understand oppression and to be able to guard against one's participation in either. Swigonski (1999) stated that "oppression and privilege are two sides of the same coin. Oppression denies individuals access to resources and opportunities as a consequence of their membership in a particular group, typically as an accident of birth. Privilege provides special access to resources and opportunities—advantages—that accrue to individuals as a consequence of their membership in a particular group, typically as an accident of birth" (Swigonski, p. 128). Admitting privilege means that one admits that discrimination exists, that one has benefited from that discrimination, and that each individual must share responsibility for discrimination. The greater the number of white people who are oblivious to white privilege, the longer racism will continue (Neville, Worthington & Spanierman, 2001). So too, the greater number of men who are oblivious to gender privilege, the longer gender discrimination will continue, the greater number of heterosexual people who are oblivious to sexual orientation privilege, the longer heterosexism will continue, and so forth.

Rejecting Privilege

Neville and colleagues (2001) point out that examining one's privileged status provides counselors with a number of benefits. According to them, counselors who are open to challenging and rejecting their own privileges are more likely to have a reduced tendency to stereotype, apply systems and contextual approaches to working with clients of color, reject culturally encapsulated counseling techniques, accept individual client worldviews, and discuss race, culture, gender, sexual orientation, and so forth with clients.

As stated previously, privilege is typically invisible to those who benefit from their privileges and acutely apparent to those who do not benefit. McIntosh (1988) has assisted many people in determining which privileges they enjoy. After reading her article, McIntosh (2004) cautions readers not to use her observations as a questionnaire, checklist, or confessional. Instead, she encourages people to make observations about their own privileges, including privileges of gender, religion, vocation, class, language, and sexual orientation. She also suggests generating answers to the following questions:

1. What is the one way you've had unearned disadvantage in your life?
2. What is one way you've had unearned advantages in your life?
3. What is it like to [express your] unearned advantages or disadvantages?

The most important question for counselors beginning to reject privilege is:

4. How can you "use unearned advantage to weaken systems of unearned advantages and why would [you] want to?"

In an effort to determine the level of awareness white counseling students possessed concerning their privileges, Ancis and Szymanski (2001) conducted a study in which white students were asked to react to Peggy McIntosh's 46 white privilege observations about herself. The students' reactions were categorized under three general themes: "Lack of awareness and denial of white privilege," (p. 554) (10 students); "Demonstrated awareness of White privilege and discrimination" (p. 557) (10 students); and "Higher order awareness and commitment to action" (p. 558) (14 students). More than a third of the students fell into the last category indicating "an awareness of the systemic nature of privilege . . . several students demonstrated an understanding of the parallels between multiple forms of oppression . . . and others took some type of action in the form of challenging their own or others' white privilege" (p. 558). Nearly another third of the students not only lacked awareness of their white privilege but expressed anger and defensiveness regarding McIntosh's list. Seven out of ten students who stated that they possessed an introductory awareness of their white privilege "either accepted no responsibility for their position or clearly indicated that they were not willing to challenge or relinquish privilege" (p. 558).

The authors expressed feelings of shock that students in a multicultural counseling class would voice such negative feelings and would be in denial of oppression. The authors were also surprised that there were so many students who were aware of the idea of "white privilege," which led the researchers to wonder whether or not the students were simply stating what they thought the instructor wanted to hear.

Overall, the study emphasizes the need for counseling students to explore white privilege as a key element in developing a non-racist identity (Ancis & Szmanski, 2001). McGrath and Axelson (1999) have devised an activity to help middle-class and able-bodied counselors experience what it is like to live without some of their privileges. For example, they suggest spending a full day in a wheelchair or not using one of your hands for a day. Similarly, the following exercise will help students begin to recognize and learn how to reject their privileges.

Exercise for Understanding Class Privilege

To simulate living in poverty, divide your living space in half and only use one half of it for the simulation. Cut your weekly budget to the bare essentials. Use no vending machines, and don't buy any unnecessary items—no gifts, no movies, no eating out at restaurants. Only use cash (no checks or credit cards), unplug your phone and put away your cell phone, give up your car, use only two or three sets of clothes, and take your clothes out to a coin laundry for washing (McGrath & Axelson, 1999). Record your experiences living in simulated poverty in the spaces below.

_____

_____

_____

_____

_____

FINAL THOUGHTS ABOUT BIASES

U.S. society has been caught in a cycle of oppression that has lasted for generations. Those who have internalized myths and misinformation about others perpetuate this cycle when they do nothing to change the cycle and pass untruths on to the next generation. The cycle can be broken if more individuals take it upon themselves to research and reject stereotypes, more people do something to fight prejudice and promote non-racist or non-oppressive practices and laws, more people choose to be open about their prejudices and racist or oppressive beliefs, and more people decide to reject rather than tacitly accept the privileges they are born with.

Unfortunately, breaking the cycle of oppression is not easy, because doing so means going against deeply enculturated beliefs. This occurs all of the time. For instance, D'Andrea and Daniels (1999) found that the white counselors, educators, graduate students, and practitioners they studied failed to act on their anti-racist beliefs to avoid negative reactions from other whites. Similarly, Neville and colleagues (2001) explored the costs of suppressing privilege, which included being ostracized for an anti-racist position, losing friends, being isolated from other whites, or being labeled a "race traitor." In addition, negative career consequences such as poor performance reviews and being refused promotions are also possible when one chooses to break the cycle of oppression. When most of a person's friends and family possess attitudes that reflect aversive racism and color-blindness, that person is unlikely to receive support or encouragement for his or her increased multicultural sensitivity.

Overcoming biases, prejudices, oppressive behavior, and privilege requires courage and perseverance. Those choosing to overcome these things will need to create coping strategies to stay on track. The following coping statements were submitted by several students as part of an exercise during a multicultural counseling course. It was at the end of the semester, and many of the students had found the class so supportive of their multicultural growth that the students wanted to create ways to maintain their awareness of cultural issues and continue to grow. The statements below constitute a "mantra" the students created so that they would not be sidetracked and retreat back into color-blindness or aversive racism.

1. I will confront the racist behaviors of my friends and relatives because I love them, and because such behaviors hurt them as well as others.
2. Possessing biases and prejudices does not make me a bad person, nor does it mean that the people I learned these biases from are bad people.
3. Unlearning biases and prejudices is difficult. It took time for me to learn all these biases and prejudices, and it will take time for me to unlearn them.
4. Before I categorically deny the truthfulness of a statement, I need to do my own research on both sides of the issue.
5. Before I categorically endorse a statement, I will do my own research on both sides of the issue.
6. If I feel angry, hurt, or sad about my beliefs and values, this is a sign that learning is beginning to occur and that I shouldn't stop learning because it feels bad. The only way to feel better is to learn more.

Creating a mantra such as this, along with a personal plan to overcome any negative consequences from your participation in oppression reduction will help you to break the cycle of oppression within yourself, within your family, and with your clients.

REVIEW/REFLECTION QUESTIONS

1. Think of some positive and negative stereotypes about your own cultural group. How difficult or burdensome would living with these stereotypes be for you? What would you do to disprove the negative stereotypes or to prove the positive ones? How do you think these stereotypes affect a person's career choices?
2. CoBRA is considered the "new racism." The essence of the argument behind CoBRA attitudes is that all people are equal. How then would one reconcile one's own CoBRA beliefs with what we have discovered about privilege?

3. It is important for counselors to learn to reject privilege to effectively work with their multicultural clients. Discuss in detail how you plan to reject privilege in your life to be more congruent as a multicultural counselor.

REFERENCES

Ancis, J. R., & Szymanski, D. M. (2001). Awareness of White privilege among White counseling trainees. *Counseling Psychologist, 29*, 548–569.

Allport, G. W. (1979). *The nature of prejudice.* Reading, MA: Addison-Wesley.

Arredondo, P., Toporek, R., Brown, S. P., Jones, J., Locke, D. C., Sanchez, J., & Stadler, H. (1996). Operationalization of the multicultural counseling competencies. *Journal of Multicultural Counseling and Development, 24*, 42–78.

Axelson, J. A. (1999). *Counseling and development in a multicultural society.* Pacific Grove, CA: Brooks/Cole Publishing Company.

Crowfoot, J. E., & Cheslery, M. A. (1996). White men's roles in multicultural coalitions. In B. J. Bowser & R. G. Hunt (Eds.), *Impacts of racism on White Americans* (2nd ed., pp. 202–229). Thousand Oaks, CA: Sage.

D'Andrea, M., & Daniels, J. (2001). Expanding our thinking about White racism: Facing the challenge of multicultural counseling in the 21st century. In J. G. Ponterotto, J. M. Casas, L. A. Suzuki & C. M. Alexander (Eds.) (pp. 289–310). *Handbook of multicultural counseling* (2nd ed.). Thousand Oaks, CA: Sage Publications.

Devine, P. G., Plant, E. A., & Buswell, B. N. (2000). Breaking the prejudice habit: Progress and obstacles (pp. 185–208). In S. Oskamp (Ed.) *Reducing prejudice and discrimination.* Mahwah, NJ: Lawrence Erlbaum Associates, Publishers.

Dovidio, J. F., Kawakami, K., & Gaertner, S. L. (2000). Reducing contemporary prejudice: Combating explicit and implicit bias at the individual and intergroup level (pp. 137–164). In S. Oskamp (Ed.) *Reducing prejudice and discrimination.* Mahway, NJ: Lawrence Erlbaum Associates, Publishers.

Haney, C., & Hurtado, A. (1994). The jurisprudence of race and meritocracy: Standardized testing and "race-neutral" racism in the workplace. *Law and Human Behavior, 18,* 223–248.

Helms, J. E., & Cook, D. A. (1999). *Using race and culture in counseling and psychotherapy: Theory and process.* Boston: Allyn and Bacon.

Jackson, R. (1999). White space, white privilege: Mapping discursive inquiry into the self. *Quarterly Journal of Speech, 85,* 35–54.

Jones, C. P. (2000). Levels of racism: A theoretic framework and a gardener's tale. *American Journal of Public Health, 90,* 1212–1215.

Jones, J. M. (1972). *Prejudice and racism.* New York: Pergamon Press.

Kincade, E., & Evans, K. (1993). *Surveying our differences: Race and women counselors.* Paper presented at the annual convention of the American Counseling Association, Atlanta, GA.

Knowles, L., & Prewitt, K. (Eds.). (1969). *Institutional racism in America.* Englewood Cliffs, NJ: Prentice-Hall.

Kovel, J. (1970). *White racism: A psychohistory.* New York: Pantheon.

McIntosh, P. (1988). *White privilege and male privilege: A personal account of coming to see correspondence through work in women's studies* (Working Paper Series No. 189). Wellesley, MA: Wellesley College, Center for Research on Women.

Neville, H. A., Worthington, R. L., & Spanierman, L. B. (2001). Counselor roles in understanding and fighting oppression. In J. G. Ponterotto, J. M. Casas, L. A. Suzuki & C. M. Alexander (Eds.) (pp. 257–288). *Handbook of multicultural counseling* (2nd ed.). Thousand Oaks, CA: Sage Publications.

Ochs, N., & Evans, K. M. (1993). How can White counselors help White clients with racial issues? In S. D. Johnson, Jr. R. Carter, E. I. Sicelides & T. R. Buckeley (Eds). *The 1993 Teachers College Winter Roundtable Conference Proceedings. Training for Competence in Cross-cultural Counseling and Psychotherapy.* New York: Teachers College, Columbia University.

Parker, W. M. (1998). *Consciousness-raising: A primer for multicultural counseling* (2nd ed.). Springfield, IL: Charles C Thomas.

Pedersen, P. (1994). *A handbook for developing multicultural awareness* (2nd ed.). Alexandria, VA: American Counseling Association.

Ponteroto, J. G., & Pedersen, P. B. (1993). *Preventing prejudice: A guide for counselors and educators.* Newbury Park, CA: Sage Publications.

Ridley, C. R. (1989). Racism in counseling as an adversive behavioral process. In P. B. Pedersen, J. G. Draguns, W. J. Lonner & J. E. Trimble (Eds.). *Counseling across cultures* (3rd ed.) (pp. 55–77).

Ridley, C. R. (1995). *Overcoming unintentional racism in counseling and therapy: A practitioner's guide to intentional intervention.* Thousand Oaks, CA: Sage Publications.

Sue, D. W., & Sue, D. (2003). *Counseling the culturally different.* New York: John Wiley & Sons, Inc.

Swigonski, M. (1999). Ways of knowing/oppression and privilege. In M. Kiselica (Ed.), *Confronting prejudice and racism during multicultural training* (pp. 123–136). Alexandria: VA: ACA.

Utsey, S. O., Bolden, M. A., & Brown, C. F. (2001). Assessing quality of life in the context of culture. In L. Suzuki & J. Ponterotto (Eds.), *Handbook of multicultural assessment: Clinical, psychological, and educational applications* (2nd ed.) (pp. 191–216). San Francisco: Jossey-Bass.

Vera, H., Feagin, J. R., & Gordon, A. (1995). Superior intellect?: Sincere fictions of the White self. *Journal of Negro Education, 64*(3), 295–306.

Wrenn, C. G. (1962). The culturally encapsulated counselor. *Harvard Educational Review, 32,* 444–449.

CHAPTER 4
Awareness of the Client's Worldview

In addition to being aware of one's cultural history and personal biases, the next most important area of multicultural competency, according to Arredondo and colleagues (1996), is the counselor's awareness of the client's worldview. Each multicultural competency is comprised of awareness, knowledge, and skill. Covered in this chapter are the awareness, knowledge, and eventual skills career counselors need to master for their culturally different clients. Research has shown that the vocational choices of ethnic minorities and other oppressed groups are influenced by a number of factors. Researchers have found that members of ethnic groups, gays and lesbians, individuals with disabilities, and others tend to gravitate toward occupations that are traditional for their groups. Reasons for this trend include an attraction by members of a group toward the historical legacy of their group's engagement in a particular occupation, an expectation of little or no discrimination in selected occupations, the avoidance of harassment or maltreatment by choosing particular professions, and family influence. A great deal of research has been conducted on the career issues facing ethnic minorities and women, especially with regard to demographic limitations placed on individuals from these groups. Less research has been done on the career issues (beyond the obvious discrimination issues) facing gay/lesbian/bisexual/transgendered persons, people with disabilities, and other non-ethnic oppressed groups, but research in these areas is ever-growing. Many of these issues will be addressed in later chapters. The primary focus of this chapter, however, will be on those factors that may influence and improve the relationship between client and counselor. The best place to start is to gain an understanding of the importance of history for ethnic minority and other oppressed clients, after which the chapter will focus on other ways in which career counselors can better gain an awareness of the needs of culturally diverse clients by understanding their worldviews. In order to understand the client's worldview, the career counselor must understand client cultural mistrust, respect client cultural expectations and values, discern differences among members of the same cultural group (within group differences), consider the client's racial/cultural development identity status, comprehend client worldview as it relates to the world of work, and understand the current political climate for culturally different clients.

UNDERSTANDING THE CLIENT'S HISTORY

In 1964, Malcolm X stated, "History is a people's memory, and without a memory, man is demoted to the lower animals." Too often counselors succumb to the temptation to disregard the cultural history of their clients. Often this is done in a futile attempt to be color blind, or blind to the client's ethnicity, religion, sexual orientation, and so forth. However, if ignoring history results in the dehumanization of a client, then a counselor can hardly be called an effective multicultural career counselor. Rather than ignore culture, an effective multicultural career counselor should respect a client's family and culture of origin. The following account of a client's experiences in therapy before this book's author became her counselor illustrates the importance of recognizing and embracing client cultural history:

Several weeks ago I went to a white female counselor who was about my age. We were getting to know one another, and I told her about my childhood escapades. I mentioned some fond memories of visiting my many relatives in Georgia. She marveled at the closeness of my extended family and offhandedly asked me how my parents could leave family behind to go to New York City. I was a little surprised by her question, but I thought I'd give her a gentle reminder. I said, "My parents left Georgia in 1957." Her reply amazed me, she asked again, "I know, but why did they leave?" I was quiet for a few moments, hoping that the shear stupidity of that question would finally dawn on her. Before I knew it, I got angry about her apparent ignorance and said, "My parents didn't want me to grow up in a place where I would be blatantly treated as a second-class citizen. They didn't want me to grow up in a place where I couldn't sit anywhere I wanted to sit on the bus or drink from any water fountain I saw. They didn't want me to grow up in a place where whites would call my father and brother 'boy' no matter how old they got and if they protested in any way they would risk being physically attached or lynched."

I was not surprised that the counselor had failed to connect the history of African American oppression in the South to the client's personal history, but I was moved by the long-lasting effect the client's experience with her insensitive counselor had upon her. It is something the client has neither forgotten nor forgiven. Counselors can avoid such blunders as not recognizing something so fundamentally obvious by learning more about the history of oppression in the United States and keeping that information in the back of their minds as they work with their clients.

Not a single minority group in the United States has escaped oppression, either at home or in the workplace. Africans were enslaved, and after the Civil War African Americans lived in a segregated America in which civil rights, including job rights, were very few; Native American Indians were murdered, uprooted, and denied access to employment; Chinese immigrants were exploited for their labor on America's railroads while being excluded from their new adopted home; Japanese Americans were taken from their homes and jobs and interned in War Relocation Camps on America's own soil during World War II; Hispanics were exploited for their labor and kept from intermingling with the dominant population; white women were denied the right to vote and prevented from entering the American workforce in all but a few professions; people with disabilities were prevented access from most public buildings and workplaces; and gay, lesbian, and bisexual individuals lived with the undesirable option of either being invisible or being visible and losing their civil rights, including the right to hold a job. It was not until the middle and late twentieth century that the United States made changes in its laws and policies, lessening the oppression of many of these groups.

Learning about the work histories of different oppressed groups lays the foundation for understanding their resentment and anger in a career counseling context. Such knowledge may also help counselors deepen their empathy towards their culturally different clients. In 2001, after the 9/11 terrorist attacks on the United States, this book's author found it interesting that her white students were completely baffled by the attack, asking, "Why do they hate us so much?" Her ethnic minority students (who were equally fearful of their safety) did not seem as baffled at the hatred. Their own anger at many of the oppressive conditions they endure every day in the United States may have allowed for a greater understanding of foreign dislike of the U.S. Career counselors who have not experienced oppression on a regular basis will need to expend a greater effort to better understand their oppressed clients.

It is beyond the scope of this work to provide a thorough history of the oppression of culturally different groups regarding work and career in the United States. However, the brief history above provides a head start. An enormous number of resources are available to inform counselors about the history, heritage, and values of specific populations as they pertain to the workplace. Volumes have been written about counseling every ethnic minority and other oppressed groups. Rather than attempt to duplicate the efforts of these many works, the focus of this section is on counselor acquisition of broad areas of knowledge applicable to all oppressed groups. Most importantly, the culturally different client's perspective of work life in the United States, as a member of an oppressed group is described in this section.

Reading history texts and biographies, and watching movies by and about members of specific oppressed groups are excellent strategies for gaining understanding and increasing empathy. Also, the Internet provides a wide range of information. It is important, however, to verify the accuracy of Internet sources. There will be sites that paint a rosy picture of a particular group and blame all problems on the dominant culture, while other sites may post jokes and present negative images and stereotypes about different groups. All of this information is useful for the counselor—even the information found on the negative sites. What better way to gain an understanding of racists, sexists, and heterosexists than to view the open hostility, hatred, and cruelty on such web sites?

There is so much information available both in print sources and on the Internet that counselors may become overwhelmed by the sheer volume of information. One may be tempted to just throw up one's hands in frustration and think that there is no way to know it all. Knowing it all, however, is *not* the goal of multicultural training, and counselors are not expected to be experts on every group. Clients are the experts on how their own group memberships have impacted their lives. Career counselors can narrow the volume of information they need by focusing on the work histories of the culturally different groups served by their schools and agencies. Also, counselors can choose not to feel overwhelmed by looking upon the gathering of information as an exciting adventure into unknown territory. The end goal is that, while they may not be able to know everything about every culture, counselors need to be able to communicate to clients that they are not ignorant about cultural issues, they care about the effect of culture on clients' lives, and they are prepared to understand clients from the clients' own perspective.

UNDERSTANDING CLIENT CULTURAL MISTRUST

Individuals who are targets of discrimination and oppression perceive events and people differently from their oppressors, which is why empathy is a critically important quality for counselors to possess. Using African Americans as the reference group, Parham and Brown (2003) noted that oppressed people "see and relate to life . . . [through lenses] colored by a set of experiences that contextualize their psychological growth and adaptation against a backdrop of socially oppressive phenomena" (p. 95). Most culturally different clients are constantly aware of how they differ from people from the dominant culture. They receive daily reminders of their differences while going about their routine tasks, and they rarely think of themselves outside the context of their own culture. It would not make sense, therefore, for counselors to decontextualize their clients' experiences by avoiding the discussion of race and culture. Equally as important as viewing the clients in the context of their culture is accepting clients' perceptions of discriminatory experiences. Truax, Cordova, Wood, Wright & Crosby (1998) stated that the targets of oppression are intimately familiar with discriminatory incidences, so it is essential for counselors to honor client assessments of oppressive incidents.

Human beings have learned to adapt to all kinds of environmental conditions, whether those conditions be geographical (for instance, adapting to harsh geographical climates), familial (such as living within a patriarchal or matriarchal family system), political (living under a dictatorship, for instance), or social. It is no wonder, then, that people would learn to deal with centuries of social oppression by developing coping strategies that over time become internalized by the cultural group. These coping strategies are passed from generation to generation, and even though the worst oppression is over for most of the groups in the United States, these coping strategies remain a part of the group culture as forms of self-protection and preservation. One of the self-protective coping strategies targets of discrimination employ in reaction to oppression is to distrust those who resemble the oppressor. Numerous studies have reported that clients generally prefer same race, same gender counselors. Coleman, Wampold, and Casali (1995) performed a meta-analysis of several studies and found that ethnic minorities prefer and rate ethnic minority counselors more highly than they rate European American counselors. "Given demographic information, potential clients will make inferences about the attitudes, values, and skills of the counselor" (p. 57). These findings seem to support the notion that clients inherently distrust cross-racial and cross-cultural counseling relationships. In other words, clients who expect to be discriminated against by European Americans are more likely to distrust European American counselors because they are members of the dominant, discriminating group (Swim, Cohen & Hyers, 1998; Baron, Burgess & Kao, 1991). Similarly, male counselors are more likely than not to be assumed to be sexist by women clients, and heterosexual counselors are more likely than not to be assumed to be heterosexist by gay/lesbian/bisexual/transgendered clients. Whaley (2001) called this phenomenon cultural mistrust. Counselors who encounter such mistrust, even hostility, from clients may be tempted to label this behavior as paranoid. Clients exhibiting such behavior may indeed be wary and suspicious, but rather than pathologize the behavior as paranoia, counselors should instead be aware that the behavior would more appropriately be defined as cultural mistrust—a realistic suspicion and lack of trust (in other words, a healthy paranoia) that is a result of ongoing, lifelong experiences with oppression (Whaley, 2001).

Further, counselors who are of the same race, culture, gender, sexual orientation, and so forth as their clients are not necessarily free from experiencing cultural mistrust from their clients. Those clients who tend to be highly mistrustful are even likely to suspect that such counselors are part of the white or dominant institution (Whaley, 2001). When counselors, regardless of background, work as part of a perceived culturally dominant institution, they may be seen by clients as having sold out their identity. Such counselors are seen as essentially the same as or even worse than counselors from the dominant group. This cultural mistrust is of the system, not necessarily of the individual counselor. Counselors would do well to become familiar with cultural mistrust and work on their own trustworthiness as multicultural counselors. Parham and Brown (2003) warn, however, that counselors can try to do what they can to show trustworthiness, but trust is more internal than external. Clients have to decide for themselves if their counselors deserve to be trusted. Counselors who reach a point of empathy with their clients, who in other words can truly put themselves in their clients' shoes and communicate this understanding to clients, are likely to break through the barrier of cultural mistrust.

Exploring Cultural Mistrust Exercise

Think of someone whom you do not trust. It may be someone who has lied to you in the past, someone who has betrayed a confidence, someone who talks behind your back, or a spouse or significant other who has cheated on you. First, list the reaction you have when you find yourself having to interact with this individual. Include in the list your feelings and your behaviors.

When I see the person I distrust I feel . . .

_____

_____

When I see the person I distrust I . . . (list things you do)

_____

_____

Next, generate a list of the things the above-mentioned person can do to regain your trust.

_____

_____

_____

_____

Many people find that the second list is a lot smaller than the first. This exercise may help you get in touch with the mistrustful feelings your culturally different clients may have toward you. In addition it gives a glimpse at how hard you may have to work to overcome this mistrust.

RESPECTING CLIENT CULTURAL EXPECTATIONS AND VALUES

When you explored your own culture in Chapter 2, you identified cultural values and expectations for your own group. A different process may be needed to determine the values and expectations of groups other than your own. You may not have easy access to the people you need to interview. Rather than interviewing relatives and friends, you may need to interview representatives of culturally different groups, such as community leaders. Identifying the expectations and values within culturally different groups helps counselors pinpoint those expectations and values that may be in conflict with their own and to resist the temptation to impose their own expectations and values onto culturally different clients. More importantly, knowledge of culturally different expectations and values will increase counselor understanding of client issues and enhance the counselor-client relationship. If, for example, research has found that a particular cultural group rejects persons of different sexual orientations, a counselor can more easily understand the point of view of a client from that cultural group who is adamant about staying in the closet in relation to his or her family. The client from that cultural group may or may not have values that match those of the counselor, but counselors must be knowledgeable about and respectful of those values nonetheless.

The expectation and value differences that seem to be particularly relevant to ethnic minority groups are those regarding family. While the dominant white Protestant middle class promotes individuality above the family, nearly all ethnic minority groups, including white ethnic groups such as Italian Americans and Irish Americans, cherish the extended family. Counselors must be familiar with the values their clients place on extended family before proceeding with counseling. The following scenario, from a high school career counselor's experience, demonstrates what can happen when counselors fail to consider the importance of family expectations and values amongst ethnic minorities during the counseling process:

I counseled Jean, a young woman from Xianggang (formerly Hong Kong), who entered counseling because she had to choose a college major and was having trouble coming up with one. She was witty, gentle, and very positive, and I enjoyed the time with her. In our third session, she confessed to me that she really wanted to become a counselor, and she said it almost apologetically. I explored with her what appealed to her about counseling, and her eyes lit up and she smiled all over. I suggested that she do some research on the counseling profession in Hong Kong—training, places of employment, and so forth. She came back the next week with a great deal of information and a lot of questions. She seemed to be a sponge—just soaking up everything she could find on the topic. I was very pleased with her progress, so it was a great surprise to me when Jean told me during our fifth session that she had changed her mind about counseling. When I asked why, she told me she had discussed the decision with her Chinese friends and her brother (who lived and worked in another state), and they told her that her English was not good enough for pursuing counseling in the United States. They advised her to stick with something they (meaning her cultural group) do well, like math or science. I could hear sadness in her voice but saw acceptance in her face. I was unaware at the time that I had mishandled Jean's counseling and that I was completely culturally insensitive. If I had it to do all over again, of course, I would have assessed her level of acculturation before embarking on an information-gathering discussion. I would have asked about the opinions of her family and significant others in her culture, and I would have explored what it would mean for her to go against her family and friends' recommendations. I know now that I will not make that kind of mistake again.

DISCERNING DIFFERENCES WITHIN THE SAME CULTURAL GROUP

Learning about the values and expectations of various cultural groups comes with a very strong caveat: Do not use this information to stereotype clients. Stereotyping has been a fear of multicultural trainers since this type of training began. Multicultural trainers feared that the counselors they trained would simply replace their uninformed stereotypes with "informed" stereotypes. This is typical behavior amongst Americans, who live in an information-heavy society and tend to convert complex ideas into simple shorthand, an example of which is the proliferation of acronyms in American speech. Even in the multicultural counseling area, the tendency to use shorthand is apparent in the use of the generic terms "African American," "Asian American," "Latino," and "Native American." When viewed critically, these terms come dangerously close to stereotyping. For example, as long as black people live in the United States, "African American" is the term that is used to describe them, whether they be U.S.-born blacks or those born in the Caribbean, South America, or Africa. Though they share racial and cultural roots as well as a common ancestry, the people of these different regions differ in a number of significant ways. Several authors have recommended being specific when referring to particular ethnic groups. For example, they have recommended that Native Americans be referred to more specifically by tribal name, that Asian Americans of Japanese descent be called Japanese American, that black Americans of Trinidadian descent be called Trinidadian Americans, and so forth.

The importance of being more specific when naming a client's ethnic group goes beyond correctness. The point is that counselors should be keenly aware of the unique within-group differences or within the culturally different groups they serve. For example, an easy way for a counselor to lose credibility with a client is for the client to perceive that the counselor believes all African Americans are the same. The counselor whose clientele includes not only individuals of African descent whose ancestors were born in the United States, but also individuals who immigrated from Haiti, Jamaica, and Aruba needs to know the cultural variations among these groups. In addition, the counselor should have an understanding of the perceptions each group has of the other groups. Nothing can be more damaging to a counseling relationship than a counselor mistaking a client's heritage for that of one of the groups his or her ethnic group despises. Further, not only do counselors need to be aware of these intragroup differences, but they must also understand that some of their clients (especially immigrants) totally reject being classified as African American, Asian American, Latino, and so forth. Take the time to know the differences within the group. Among the within-group differences that have the most profound affects on the counseling relationship are those related to racial and cultural identity. But note also that people from other oppressed groups are not all the same. For example, women differ (among other factors) in terms of race/ethnicity/culture, age, and marital status; people with disabilities differ in terms of types of disability—motor, visual, hearing impairment, psychological; and though they tend to be identified as one group gay men differ from lesbians, and they both differ from bisexual and transgendered individuals. Counselors must demonstrate an ability to see within-group differences.

Within-Group Differences Exercise

Listed below are the cultural groups that are the focus of this text. Under each group, generate as many subgroups that you can think of. For example, a few subgroups of African Americans have already been mentioned (African-born, Caribbean-born). Try not to limit your list to geography—think of all the areas of culture that may diversify a group (religion—such as Irish Catholics and Irish Protestants, language).

African Americans

_____

_____

_____

American Indian/Alaska Native

_____

_____

_____

Asian American

_____

_____

_____

Latinos and Latinas

_____

_____

_____

People with Disabilities

_____

_____

_____

Gays, Lesbians, Bisexual, and Transgendered Individuals

_____

_____

_____

White Women

_____

_____

_____

CONSIDERING THE CLIENT'S RACIAL/CULTURAL IDENTITY DEVELOPMENT STATUS

In Chapter 2, you became more aware of your own racial/cultural values, expectations, and traditions, and how you have internalized (or not internalized) those aspects of your identity. As discussed in that chapter, this is referred to as your racial/cultural identity development stage or status. Racial/cultural identity development stage/status is as relevant to clients as it is to counselors. For example, an Asian American counselor assigned to a white client whose racial identity development stage is reintegration may have trouble with a client disdainful of other races and cultures, as is characteristic of the reintegration stage. Similarly, an Asian American client at the conformity stage of racial/cultural identity development may resent and resist an Asian American counselor, because a rejection of one's own race is characteristic of the conformity stage. For another example, consider the importance of being aware of the racial/cultural identity development stage in the following counseling scenario, in which the client is clearly in the resistance stage of development:

Starr Adams is an African American high school counselor whose primary duties involve offering career counseling to the students. Star's first client was a nineteen-year-old Mexican American female, Patricia, who was openly hostile to Starr and requested that a Latina counselor work with her. Patricia stated further that the counseling center was racist because they gave all the minority students to Starr no matter their race or ethnicity, and the white kids and black kids got to work with counselors who look like them but the Latinos/as had to settle for whoever was in the office. She also voiced the opinion that the white counselors didn't want to be bothered with the Latinos or blacks and didn't care what kind of service they got. Starr was devastated by Patricia's attitude and was clueless about what she should do. She didn't even get a chance to establish rapport, credibility, or trust.

As the above scenario demonstrates, counselors who rightfully approach the counseling situation with the notion that they must clearly demonstrate their own acceptance of racially and culturally different clients often fail to consider that due to the client's racial identity development stage, the client may reject the counselor simply because of the counselor's race or culture. Therefore, the counselor who is able to assess a client's racial identity development stage and work with the client from wherever the client may be on the continuum is more likely to be successful and culturally competent than the counselor who does not have such expertise. In the above scenario, the hostile client in the resistance stage might more effectively be referred to a European American counselor whose own racial/cultural identity development is of a higher status level. This is just what Helms (1990) and Helms and Cook (1999) have suggested—that effective counselors must function at higher racial/cultural identity development stages/statuses than those of their clients. These authors (1999) presented a model that illustrates the interactions both between counselors and their supervisors and between group leaders and group members based on racial/cultural identity development stage/status. Although the Helms and Cook model focused on a supervisor/worker relationship, a similar process occurs between client and counselor. In fact, Helms states, "I originally proposed . . . and continue to believe that racial identity models will make it feasible to train therapists who can be responsive to intrapersonal as well as interpersonal racial dynamics both within and outside the therapy relationship" (p. 196). Helms described the interactions between two people (dyads) such as a counselor and a client (Helms, 1990) and devised four different relationship types based on the racial/cultural identity development stage/status of both the client and the counselor. Helms suggests that regardless of the number of people involved, the relationships are always progressive, parallel, regressive, or crossed.

The ideal counseling relationship is the progressive relationship. In a progressive counseling relationship, the counselor's racial identity status is at least one level higher than that of the client, and the counselor is therefore able to facilitate client growth. For example, the white counselor at the Pseudo-Independent status (the status wherein an intellectual understanding of racial/cultural differences has developed) can be in a progressive counseling relationship if the client is in the contact stage (the stage wherein the client is naïve about racism and other cultural groups). This relationship is productive and beneficial to the client (Helms, 1990).

The parallel relationship occurs when the client and counselor see the world in the same way. For example, a parallel relationship would be one in which a white counselor in the contact status, who, as characteristic of this status, sees no need to change the status quo, works with an ethnic minority client who is in the conformity stage and, as characteristic of that stage, thinks that racism does not exist and that the status quo is acceptable. There is little chance of conflict in a parallel relationship, because the goal for both the client and the counselor is to avoid conflict and tension (Helms, 1990). However, there is also little chance for growth on the part of the client or the counselor.

In regressive relationships, the client's racial/cultural identity development is at a higher stage than that of the counselor. Take for example an ethnic minority client who is at the Integrative stage of racial/cultural identity development (characterized by appreciating one's own group and other groups) meeting a counselor who is at the Immersion status (characterized as a white person intensively trying to understand why white people don't work hard enough correcting their racist attitudes). In the above relationship, there is little that the counselor can do to help the client grow and develop culturally, since the client has already worked through his or her issues with race/culture. In fact, the client, who is the one seeking help, is more sophisticated regarding race/culture than the counselor. This type of relationship is likely to be strained and unproductive (Helms, 1990).

The final relationship, the crossed relationship, is the most troublesome. These types of relationships are most likely to fail because the racial/cultural identity development stages/statuses of the client and the counselor are diametrically opposed. The client and counselor hold "opposing attitudes towards Blacks and Whites" (p. 141). Helms states that these types of dyads are "antagonistic and short-lived" (p. 195). For example, the ethnic minority counselor is in the conformity stage while the white client is in the autonomy stage.

Whatever the relationship type, for both the client and the counselor, racial identity reflects the individual's way of coping with racism in U.S. society and contributes significantly to his or her worldviews—worldviews that include how they perceive the world of work.

Counseling Relationship Dyads Exercise

Identify the following Counseling Dyads as Parallel, Progressive, Regressive, or Crossed.

Counselor	Client	
Conformity	Pseudo-Independent	_____
Disintegration	Dissonance	_____
Autonomy	Introspection	_____
Resistance	Reintegration	_____

COMPREHENDING CLIENT WORLDVIEW AS IT RELATES TO THE WORLD OF WORK

As noted in Chapter 2, Sue and Sue (2003) describe worldview using the locus of control and locus of responsibility paradigms. As you may recall, the locus of control pertains to whether or not people believe they have control over factors in their lives and the locus of responsibility pertains to whether or not people believe they are responsible for the things that happen in their lives. Please refer back to Figure 2.1 in Chapter 2 for an illustration of these concepts. As you can see, Sue and Sue placed the locus of control and locus of responsibility perpendicularly on a continuum, resulting in four quadrants. Career counselors who comprehend where their clients fall within these four quadrants will be better able to help their clients in the career counseling process.

Quadrant I—Internal Locus of Control and Internal Locus of Responsibility

The first quadrant is most descriptive of European American middle-class culture. Individuals with an internal locus of control and an internal locus of responsibility believe that they are responsible for whatever successes they achieve and failures they experience. They also believe that they have the ability to attain success on their own merits and that no one has greater control over their lives than they do. The other three quadrants explain the various worldviews of ethnic minority and oppressed group members.

Quadrant II—External Locus of Control and Internal Locus of Responsibility

Quadrant II represents the first minority worldview. Individuals who perceive the world from this perspective tend to resemble those whose racial/cultural identity development is in the conformity stage. Individuals in this quadrant hold a negative view of those in their own racial/cultural group and believe that the problems of the group, such as difficulties locating and/or sustaining employment, are due to their own shortcoming, rather than blaming oppression. In counseling, these clients tend to give full credibility to their counselor only if the counselor is a member of the dominant cultural group. Counselors from the dominant group, therefore, must be careful to properly manage the power clients hand over to them. Ethnic minority counselors, on the other hand, need to work harder at credibility and building trust.

Quadrant III—External Locus of Control and an External Locus of Responsibility

Clients in this category can prove to be a challenge to counseling professionals because these clients take no responsibility for their actions and believe that they have no control over their own lives. In other words, clients with this worldview suffer from what has been coined learned helplessness—they have tried and failed so many times that they stop trying. These clients sincerely believe that no matter what they do, nothing changes and that someone or some institution will make all of the major decisions in their lives. Such clients are difficult to motivate into the world of work or into a career change, because they do not believe that they have any power over their own lives.

Quadrant IV—Internal Locus of Control with an External Locus of Responsibility

This quadrant represents the healthiest of the minority worldviews. Individuals with this type of worldview believe that there are oppressed groups who are discriminated against and who are treated unfairly. But these individuals also believe that they can succeed on their own merits when discrimination is taken out of the equation (Sue & Sue, 2003). These clients are likely to be distrustful of counselors from the dominant culture. As a result, counselors from the dominant culture will be required to prove their competence. If dominant culture career counselors expect the Quadrant IV clients to take all the responsibility for changes in their work lives, the counseling relationship will be strained or, perhaps, prematurely terminated. These clients believe that it is the system that is broken and needs changing, not themselves. The counselor who is able to empathize with these clients and see the world from their eyes will be more successful than the counselor who doesn't comprehend what "the system" means.

UNDERSTANDING THE CURRENT POLITICAL CLIMATE FOR ETHNIC MINORITIES

Lastly, multiculturally competent counselors must be aware of the social and political influences affecting ethnic minority and other oppressed clients. Racism, sexism, ableism, heterosexism, and other "isms" oppress groups to the point that they become victims. Ridley (1995) explains that victims suffer from feelings of shame, self-blame, rage, vulnerability, and violation. What is worse, as Ridley contends, "many victims, because their feelings are unresolved, continue to play the victim role . . . [and] when victimization is selective and repeated, it is not just victimization, [targets are] singled out for who they are to inflict harm on them" (p. 5). In other words, when a person is subjected to oppression on a continuous basis, significant psychological harm often results—harm that the mental health system can sometimes contribute to as well; even in counseling and psychotherapy, clients are victimized. They are frequently misdiagnosed, their symptoms are often ignored or minimized, and they are regularly patronized (Ridley, 1995). Clients who have experienced any or all of these situations may enter counseling with negative expectations and will likely be suspicious of and uncooperative with their counselors.

The sociopolitical reality for oppressed groups is that there are systems in place that limit their potential, erect barriers for them, and deny them privileges. These discriminatory institutional policies exist at the local, state, federal, and private levels. All effective counselors need to stay current about the policies, procedures, and laws that affect their clients. Multiculturally competent counselors must go a step further and be watchful for the political realities that are especially relevant to their clients from oppressed groups. Still further, knowledge is not enough. Effective multiculturally competent counselors must also be advocates for their clients. Social injustices are often as responsible for client issues as the client's behavior. It would be rather short-sighted for counselors to assume that changing the client's behavior alone will rectify the injustices he or she has experienced.

Some recent federal laws particularly relevant to multicultural career counseling are the Civil Rights Act of 1964 and 1991, the Americans with Disabilities Act of 1990, the Welfare Reform Bill of 1996, and the Equal Pay Act of 1963, among others, which will be described in detail below. Most of these measures have proved to be beneficial for many oppressed populations. Although none of them have eliminated oppression altogether, these laws have provided some relief and can be considered moves in the right direction. From a counseling perspective, counselors should consider that, while the existence of these laws may not be felt in the everyday lives of clients, counselors may be able to use their knowledge of the laws to empower their clients and support the notion that client problems are not all of their own making. These laws represent the fact that there really are powerful forces working against people but that sometimes people can fight against those in power and effect positive changes.

The Civil Rights Act

The law with the most sweeping changes, of course, was the Civil Rights Act of 1964, which was designed to eliminate discrimination. Ethnic minority group members and white women were able to enter professions they never believed they could enter. However, during the 1980s, the Supreme Court handed down some decisions that effectively wiped out advances already gained through the Civil Rights Act. For example, the court's rulings made it difficult for plaintiffs to receive monetary compensation for discrimination, because the burden of proof was placed upon them to prove employer discrimination. Fortunately, in 1991, a new Civil Rights law overturned the earlier court decision. Under the new Civil Rights Act, the plaintiff is entitled to monetary damages for pain and suffering and economic loss resulting from the discriminatory acts of the defendant, and the burden of proof that the discrimination did not occur is now upon the defendant.

Affirmative Action

The original Civil Rights Act in 1964 led to the development of Affirmative Action, a policy that sought to redress past discrimination through active equal opportunity measures, for instance companies actively recruiting women into jobs traditionally held only by men, such as jobs in engineering. Today, however, Affirmative Action faces the same uphill battle once faced by the Civil Right Act itself. The objections to Affirmative Action range from the accusation that it is reverse discrimination to the claim that Affirmative Action is psychologically harmful to its beneficiaries. While claims of reverse discrimination may come from traditionally privileged populations, the psychological harm theory is focused on the beneficiaries of Affirmative Action. The claim posits that these beneficiaries may believe that others will "question their competence . . . which would then lower self-esteem" (Truax et al., 1998, p. 171). Steele (1991) assumed that an individual's hiring into a job via Affirmative Action would result in that individual feeling stigmatized. This assumption has not held up under research. Several studies (Ayers, 1992; Taylor, 1994; Truax et al., 1998) found that Affirmative Action hiring created "positive rather than negative effects for one minority group" (Truax et al., 1998, p. 178) and that any stigma was not related specifically to Affirmative Action but public opinion of Affirmative Action hires. In fact,

Gallup (1995) reported that fewer than 30 percent of the ethnic minority respondents polled seemed to be worried about any perceived negative consequences of being hired through Affirmative Action. Therefore, it seems that shame and embarrassment are not the emotions attached to being hired through Affirmative Action.

However helpful Affirmative Action has been, its effects have not reached out to all oppressed groups. Research shows that the two populations that have benefited most from Affirmative Action are white women and middle-class African Americans. Few poor ethnic minorities have been able to cross the cultural divide of race and poverty. Middle-class African Americans are most likely to be acculturated to the middle-class societal structure, and as such they are more readily accepted by institutions of higher education, business, and industry. In addition, middle-class African Americans have at their disposal more resources that contribute positively to their career aspirations and educational advances. These same hypotheses could be made regarding middle-class white women. More remedies are needed to cover the other oppressed groups more effectively.

The Americans with Disabilities Act

Affirmative Action also has not been as helpful as it might have been for individuals with disabilities, which is why the Americans with Disabilities Act (ADA) was created. The ADA was a major political feat for people with disabilities. It was passed in 1990 and took effect in 1992. The goal of the act was to eliminate hiring discrimination against people with disabilities in both private companies and government. In addition, the ADA prohibits discrimination in all other areas of employment, such as insurance coverage and other benefits. Finally, the ADA requires not only employers but also public facilities to make accommodations for people with disabilities, including accessible transportation.

Gay, Lesbian, Bisexual, and Transgender Rights

The Civil Rights Acts of 1964 and 1991 and Affirmative Action do not protect gays or lesbians, or bisexual and transgendered individuals from discrimination of any sort. However, during the Clinton administration, the president issued an Executive Order regarding the treatment of federal employees, which stated that there would no longer be discrimination based on sexual orientation. While this was not a law and offered no new expressed civil rights to gays and lesbians, the order set a precedent for considering sexual orientation in future antidiscrimination policies. Interestingly, gay white males enjoy the highest incomes of any of the oppressed groups, but because of the limits on discrimination laws, their incomes may come at the price of being closeted to their colleagues and superiors in the workplace. Discrimination against gay, lesbian, bisexual, and transgendered populations is not illegal, but the ethics and morality of oppressing any group for any reason is suspect.

Women's Rights

Women of all races were slotted to benefit from the Equal Pay Act of 1963. It provided that individuals doing the same job for the same company would earn the same amount of money. Under this legislation employers are not allowed to reduce the pay of men in order to comply with the law. Even with this law in place, however, women are still earning less than men for the same work (Herlihy & Watson, 2006). Apparently, employers seem to have circumvented this legislation since wage disparities between men and women still exist.

Another law that has benefited working women was Title VII of the Civil Rights Act of 1964, which stated in one of its provisions that sexual harassment is a form of discrimination, and that an employer cannot fire or demote an employee who sues due to the violation of this law.

Additionally, a positive legislative act that has benefited both female and male workers is the Family Leave Act, which made it possible for individuals to take time off from work to provide for their families without losing their jobs doing so. This legislation is especially helpful for single parents (overwhelmingly female, and overrepresented in ethnic minority groups). The Family Leave Act is a first step towards a better lifestyle for workers. The act does not require that employees be paid for the time loss, but there is a guarantee that the employee may return to his or her job after taking the leave.

The Welfare Reform Bill

On the negative side of the coin, the Welfare Reform Bill of 1996 made sweeping changes to the welfare system and impacted immigrants negatively. Not only did it cut off assistance for illegal immigrants, but it also eliminated benefits for *legal* immigrants. Those who have legally immigrated to the United States can no longer receive food stamps, nor do they receive supplemental social security benefits if they are disabled. It is legislation that seems to put undue hardship on the poor immigrants of this country. So far, Congress has not renewed the Welfare Reform bill, but neither has it terminated the bill's practices. The renewal is, at this writing, still being debated in Congress.

Poverty

Along with legislation affecting ethnic minorities and other oppressed groups, multiculturally responsible career counselors should be aware of another major political issue in American society today: poverty.

In 1999, 12.4 percent of the US population lived at or below the poverty line. Ethnic minority groups have continued to be overrepresented among the poor. The tendency in the past was for writers and researchers to combine race/ethnicity and poverty in their findings. Unfortunately, by collapsing these categories precious data has been lost at best, and the worst case scenario is that inaccurate assumptions have been made based on the results of this flawed methodology. Even though the majority of ethnic minority families are *not* classified as poor, their numbers among the poor, in general, are far greater than the 8.1 percent of whites living in poverty. Almost 25.7 percent of Native Americans/Alaska Natives live at or below the poverty line as well as 25 percent of African Americans, 22.6 percent of Latinos and Latinas, and 12.6 percent of Asian Americans.

What is really tragic is that many people who are poor actually have jobs. This has become such a prevalent phenomenon that a term has been coined to describe these individuals—the working poor (Rank, 2000). People who are poor, regardless of race, present a dilemma for the career counselor. Individuals living in poverty often do not see the relevance of career counseling, because their focus is on making enough money to pay for food, clothing, and shelter. Making career choices also becomes irrelevant when one has limited education and limited prospects for increasing one's educational level. Clients who come from generations of poverty may be particularly wary of counselors, who they believe may look down on them and their lifestyle. It is unlikely that the poor would seek career counseling on their own. They are more likely to become clients if they have lost their jobs, become part of the welfare to work initiative, or experienced some other time-sensitive program. If a working poor client is also struggling to survive, dealing with an employer's discriminatory policies, completing demeaning job duties, or facing problems either of intolerance or invisibility from co-workers, the counseling problems are magnified. Similarly, clients who are unemployed have multiple issues. While unemployment affects all socioeconomic levels, it is more likely to result in homelessness when it occurs to those who are already poor. In 2001, overall unemployment was 4.8 percent while it was 6.6 percent for Hispanics and 8.7 percent for African Americans. Besides needing to find a job, unemployed clients are most likely angry, grieving, ashamed, and doubtful of their own abilities (Evans, 2006).

Poor and unemployed clients may view counseling with desperation (a last chance) or as too little to late. It is also likely that after a long relationship with the bureaucracy, they will have little faith in their employment counselor's ability to help them with their problems. The client may take one look at his or her middle-class counselor and determine that the counselor would have no earthly idea how to help. The counselor may be resented if change does not happen quickly or if the counselor does not take time to establish credibility and trustworthiness. Therefore counselors need to be aware not only of the existence of and ramifications of poverty, but also of community resources and information they should have readily available.

FINAL THOUGHTS ABOUT CLIENT WORLDVIEW

Because career counselors serve as a gateway to a client's livelihood and lifestyle, awareness of the client's worldview is imperative because awareness can increase the length of time a client stays in counseling, drawing greater benefit from the process. Oppression has had a detrimental effect on ethnic minorities, white women, gays, lesbians, bisexuals, trangendered persons, and people with disabilities. Because of oppression, counselors, who may simply desire to help others, may be resented and treated as the enemy. It is really important for counselors to be prepared for any negative reactions that their clients may have. Rather than taking these reactions personally, counselors must learn to cope with such responses. Knowledge of the client's cultural history can go a long way in understanding client reactions to the dominant culture and may also increase the counselor's empathy toward the client's cultural group. Client racial/cultural identity status helps the counselor understand more about how to manage the counseling relationship as does the client's view of his or her locus of control and locus of responsibility. Finally, knowledge of the effects of poverty and socio-political oppression helps the career counselor encourage proactive measures in the client and commit to doing more herself or himself.

All the above factors translate into a counselor's genuine interest in the client's success and well-being. When a counselor is genuinely interested in his or her clients, the clients will know and they are likely to respond positively to the counselor and the counseling process.

REVIEW/REFLECTION QUESTIONS

1. A client who is culturally different from you is being openly hostile when you try to help her define her particular career problem. Discuss
   (a) your feelings regarding the treatment the client is giving you,
   (b) strategies you can use to depersonalize the client's attack,
   (c) how you would respond to such a client.
2. Affirmative Action, the ADA, and the Pay Equity legislation affect career counseling more than almost any other field of counseling. Discuss your attitudes and beliefs about these laws and policies. Also, discuss how your attitudes may affect your work with clients protected by these practices.
3. The knowledge of the history of the career development of culturally diverse clients is stressed in the chapter. It is a step that many counselors like to skip. How would you go about motivating yourself to explore the work histories of the client populations you serve or will serve?
4. The dominant middle-class perspective on work and getting ahead can be a detriment when working with clients who have only known poverty. It may be one of the most difficult differences for career counselors to understand. List five strategies that would be helpful in understanding a life of poverty.

REFERENCES

Arredondo, P., Toporek, R., Brown, S. P., Jones, J., Locke, D. C., Sanchez, J., & Stadler, H. (1996). Operationalization of the multicultural counseling competencies. *Journal of Multicultural Counseling and Development, 24*, 42–78.

Ayers, L. (1992). Perceptions of affirmative action among its beneficiaries. *Social Justice Research, 5*, 223–238.

Baron, R. S., Burgess, M. L., & Kao, C. F. (1991). Detecting and labeling prejudice: Do female perpetrators go undetected? *Personality and Social Psychology Bulletin, 17*, 115–123.

Coleman, H. L. K., Wampold, B. E., & Casali, S. L. (1995). Ethnic minorities' ratings of ethnically similar and European American counselors: A meta-analysis. *Journal of Counseling Psychology, 42, 55*–64.

Evans, K. M. (2006). Career counseling with couples and families. In D.Capuzzi & M. Staufer (Eds.). *Career and Life Style Planning: Theory and Application* (pp. 336–359). Boston: Pearson Education, Inc.

Gallup Short Subjects (July, 1995). *Gallup Poll Monthly, 358,* 34–61.

Helms, J. E. (1990). *Black and White racial identity: Theory, research, and practice.* New York: Greenwood Press.

Helms, J. E., & Cook, D. A. (1999). *Using race and culture in counseling and psychotherapy: Theory and process.* Boston: Allyn and Bacon.

Herlihy, B. R., & Watson, Z. P. (2006). Gender issues in career counseling. In D. Capuzzi & M. Staufer (Eds.). *Career and Life Style Planning: Theory and Application* (pp. 363–385). Boston: Pearson Education, Inc.

Parham, T. A., & Brown, S. (2003). Therapeutic approaches with African American Populations. In Harper, F. D. & McFadden, J. (Eds.) *Culture and Counseling: New approaches* (pp. 81–98). Needham Heights, MA: Allyn & Bacon.

Rank, M. R. (2000). Poverty and hardship in families. In D. H. Demo, K. R. Allen, & M. A. Fine (Eds.). *Handbook of family diversity* (pp. 293–315). New York: Oxford University Press.

Ridley, C. R. (1995). *Overcoming unintentional racism in counseling and therapy: A practitioner's guide to intentional intervention.* Thousand Oaks, CA: Sage Publications.

Steele, S. (1991). *The content of our character.* New York: St. Martin's Press.

Sue, D. W., & Sue, D. (2003). *Counseling the culturally different.* New York: John Wiley & Sons, Inc.

Swim, J. K., Cohen, L. L., & Hyers, L. L. (1998). Experiencing everyday prejudice and discrimination. In J. K. Swim, & C. Stangor, C. (Eds.), Prejudice*: The target's perspective* (38–61). San Diego: Academic Press.

Taylor, M. E. (1994). Affirmative Action: Insights from social psychological and organizational research. *Basic and Applied Social Psychology, 15,* 1–21.

Truax, K., Cordova, D. I., Wood, A., Wright, E., & Crosby, F. (1998). Undermined? Affirmative action from the target's point of view. In J. K. Swim, & C. Stangor, C. (Eds.) Prejudice*: The target's perspective* (172–188). Sand Diego, CA: Academic Press.

Whaley, A. L. (2001). Cultural mistrust and mental health services for African Americans: A review and meta-analysis. *Counseling Psychologist, 29,* 513–521.

CHAPTER 5
Using Career Development Theories

To be useful in the real world, a theory has to pass certain tests. One of the tests of the effectiveness of a counseling theory is whether or not the theory is comprehensive. The traditional career development theories tend to fall short of comprehensiveness, because they describe the behaviors of a specific group of people (typically white males) rather than a broad range of people. As Gottfredson (1986) and Leong (1995) have both said, "there is yet to appear a detailed description and explanation of how political, social, economic, and cultural conditions affect individuals and their career choice behavior" (p. 143). Picking up from where Gottfredson and Leong left off, Neville, Gysbers, Heppner, and Johnston (1998) identified five main problems with the traditional career development theories:

1. They place great significance on the individual without mention of others involved in the career decision-making process;
2. They assume that clients are at least at a middle-class socioeconomic level and that clients can therefore afford to take advantage of training opportunities;
3. They assume that work is freely available for those who want it;
4. They assume that work is of equal importance in everyone's life; and
5. They depend on linear and objective reasoning.

As alluded to above, the most troubling shortcoming of the traditional career-development theories is that despite extensive research on career development that has accompanied these theories, little evidence exists that proves or disproves that the theories are appropriate for all groups of people (Leong, 1995). In some studies, the research has proven a theory to be cross-cultural, while in other studies the results have been either contradictory or inconclusive. The bottom line is that just about every career development text mentions that the traditional career development theories are suspect when applied to ethnic minority populations and other oppressed groups. Career development theorists themselves acknowledge the importance of considering matters not under the control of clients, such as oppression and socioeconomic factors, when developing career theories. More recent theories have tended to allow for the fact that societal restrictions have a strong impact on the career choices and advancement of many individuals.

In this chapter, the traditional career theories still widely used today will be presented followed by some suggestions for adapting these theories to multicultural populations. Some recent, more multiculturally inclusive theories will then be discussed. The chapter will conclude with three current career counseling models that were designed to provide guidelines for practice with diverse populations.

THE TRADITIONAL CAREER DEVELOPMENT THEORIES

As discussed in the opening paragraphs of this chapter, most of the traditional career development theories fall short of taking into consideration political, social, economic, and cultural factors that affect clients from diverse, oppressed populations. The traditional theories covered in this chapter include Parsons' trait and factor theory, Super's career development theory, Holland's personality types and environments theory, and Krumboltz's social learning theory of career development.

Frank Parsons' Trait and Factor Theory   1909

No discussion of career development theory would be complete without reference to trait and factor theory. It was founded on the propositions of Frank Parsons in 1909. The essence of the theory is that it posits that individuals possess measurable traits and abilities that can be matched with occupational requirements. When the match is appropriate, the result is a life of occupational satisfaction and productivity for an individual.

In its early days, traditional trait and factor counseling extensively utilized paper and pencil inventories to assess client interests, values, personality, aptitudes, and abilities (Sharf, 2002). Upon completion of the inventories, clients would have objective information about their traits, which they could compare with job specifications.

However, as simple and useful as trait and factor inventories sound, multicultural theorists have criticized trait and factor theory's overdependence on measurement methods that don't take into consideration norms (standard patterns of behavior) for culturally different groups. Rather, only the norms of the dominant white, middle-class, male, heterosexual group are taken into consideration (Fouad, 1993). Because of the lack of norms for diverse groups in trait and factor theory, the theory forces a career counselor to compare a culturally different client to a set of norms that may not apply. Fouad therefore suggests that until norms for culturally different clients are developed, counselors should use caution. Some career test publishers are becoming more responsive to this problem. For example, the 1994

[handwritten margin notes:]
Traits - Characteristics of an individual

Factors - Characteristics of work environment

Matching Theories = Measure who person in or what work environment is, in the moment, in a static way.

Its "A good Match"

Traits ←——→ Factors
  to know   Can measure

Traits
- Values
- Skills
~ Interests
- abilities
- aptitudes

(qualitative)
*work ethic

JDS = interests
       & personality

Myers-Briggs = Personality

at core personality
is not changeable

ASVAB - skills/abilities

Parson's Theory
① know yourself
② know the world of
    work
③ "True reasoning"
   on these two sets
   of facts.

revision of the Strong Interest Inventory considered race and ethnicity for the first time by reporting the race and ethnicity of the comparison groups.

Fouad has pointed out another problem with trait and factor theory as it relates to culturally different populations. The problem is the use of language in trait and factor testing. Counselors should always ask, "Is the test written in the language most appropriate for the testee?" If not, then counselors should seriously consider whether or not the test should be administered.

In addition, Prince, Uemura, Chao, and Gonzalez (1991) have suggested that some cultural groups do not benefit from the introspective behaviors required in trait and factor inventories, and therefore it would be inappropriate to administer these tests to these clients.

Finally, Leong and Serafica (2001) have questioned whether the traits that have been determined by trait and factor testing to fit certain occupations are the same for all racial groups. Leong and Serafica suggest that the traits that are considered important for European American men to perform a particular job well might be considered inappropriate for Latinos and Latinas or white women. For example, competitiveness is considered an admirable trait for white men in some occupations, but competitiveness in women in that same occupation is still looked upon negatively. Or there may be separate criteria to enter an occupation for ethnic minorities and other oppressed groups—criteria that cannot be determined through objective testing. Because of discrimination and oppression, even if clients have the stated traits needed for the job, they may not be satisfied and happy in the career because of unspoken criteria.

In trait and factor counseling, clients are the ones who must find information about careers, not counselors, which means clients must not only understand how the job-finding process works, but also understand the specific abilities they possess, and the specific responsibilities various jobs entail. The creation of the O*Net database has made this process much easier than it used to be. Clients can enter O*Net from the Department of Labor's web site and access the worker attributes and job characteristics by clicking a button (*http://online.onetcenter.org*).

After clients receive information about their "traits," they need to match their traits with the occupations that require those traits. Matching (that is helping individuals find fitting careers) is the ultimate goal of all career counseling. Therefore trait and factor theory must move with the times to take into consideration culturally different clients, if counselors are to be able to use trait and factor theory to help clients locate work.

Trait and factor theory has of course evolved since 1909. Today, trait and factor counselors are less likely to rely only on test scores to predict career choices, and they are more likely to consider other factors that contribute to client decision making. Trait and factor approaches such at the Person/Environment Fit is an example of this type of evolution. Other adaptations of trait and factor theory will be discussed below.

Adapting Trait and Factor Theory for Diverse Clients

In 2001, Leong and Serafica devised a list of "cultural accommodations" that should be implemented to extend trait and factor theory to help ethnic minority and other oppressed clients. These cultural accommodations consist of a three-step process:

1. Identifying the cultural gaps or cultural blind spots of the theory
2. Selecting current culturally specific concepts and models from cross-cultural and ethnic minority psychology to fill in the gaps and adapt the theory for racial/cultural minorities
3. Testing the culturally adapted theory to determine whether or not it has incremental validity above and beyond the culturally unadapted theory (p. 185)

As stated previously, what is missing in the trait and factor theory is both an understanding that certain traits desirable for one group may not be as desirable for other groups, and a realization that there is no way to determine test bias if test publishers do not include normative samples for ethnic minority and other oppressed groups in their reports.

In adapting trait and factor theory to work more appropriately for ethnic minority and other oppressed groups, the concept of cultural encapsulation should be kept in mind. The assumption that what is good for one group is good for all groups is cultural encapsulation. Therefore, counselors need to forewarn their clients that information on traits that particular occupations require may in fact differ from one racial group to another. In addition, counselors and clients need to do the research to find out the cultural biases that exist toward the client's group within a particular profession.

Counselors themselves will demonstrate that they are culturally encapsulated if they use tests that are based on norms for white European Americans without regard to the possibility that the norms of the test may not be applicable to other groups. Counselors, therefore, should always determine if the tests they use are culturally sensitive. In summary, the trait and factor theory may be useful as it exists if counselors are extremely cautious about using tests that fail to report norms for culturally different groups or if counselors are willing and able to collect their own data to create local norms for tests that are culturally encapsulated and use those norms when interpreting client scores.

Personal Career Assessment Exercise

Make a list of your ten most outstanding characteristics (such as outgoing, witty, thoughtful, creative).

_____

_____

_____

Think of the careers you thought you wanted to pursue when you were ten years old. Chose one of the careers, different from the one you are now pursuing, and list the characteristics you believe would be required in that career.

_____

_____

_____

How well do the two lists match up? Do you think you would be successful and happy in that career? Why or why not? Finally create a list of characteristics required by your present career (or one you seek to enter).

How does that list measure up to your own personality characteristics? Do you believe that you will be happy and successful in that career if the two lists did not match? Why or why not?

Donald Super's Career Developmental Theory

Perhaps the most comprehensive, well-researched career counseling theory continues to be the career developmental theory of Donald Super. In his theory, Super (1957) described the processes individuals employ to learn about, gain, maintain, and leave their careers. Super explains that the primary purpose for choosing a career is fulfillment of one's self-concept. Factors that influence the fulfillment of self-concept are life span and life space, which will be discussed in more detail below.

Fulfillment of Self-Concept

Super (1957) originally proposed that each occupation defines a unique role for its occupants. That occupation is chosen on the basis of perceived compatibility of that role with the individual's self-concept. The self-concept may be defined as the perception individuals have of themselves combined with how others perceive them. Unfortunately, proof that Super's theory is applicable to diverse groups has been elusive. The fulfillment of self-concept theory has been questioned in regard to ethnic minorities and other oppressed groups because discrimination and poverty may prohibit individuals from fulfilling their self-concepts through work. Except for the fact that work provides the income for life's necessities, work is not a salient aspect of many minority individuals' lives (Murray et al., 2002).

Life Span

The "life span" segment of the theory involves career maturity, or an individual's readiness to move through the stages of career development based on his or her age. Super's (1957) Career Pattern Study pinpointed these stages of career development as the growth stage, the exploration stage, the establishment stage, the maintenance stage, and the disengagement stage. In the growth stage, a person develops a sense of self and identity and gains an understanding of the world of work. During the exploration stage, an individual crystallizes and implements a career choice. In the establishment stage, the individual stabilizes, consolidates, and moves up the career ladder. During the maintenance stage, the individual holds on to his or her place in the organization by updating skills or reinventing the career to fit his or her life better. Finally, in the disengagement stage, the individual plans for retirement, reduces pace and/or workload, and eventually engages in full-time leisure activities.

Originally Super presented these stages as age-specific, with growth ending at age fourteen and maintenance ending at age sixty-four. In subsequent discussions of his theory, Super responded to one of the major changes that had occurred in society since he originally mapped out the theory—that individuals no longer typically stay in the same careers their entire lives, as was once common. Super came to recognize that when changing careers, individuals go through much the same process as they did when they chose a career the first time, and that the career development process continues in cycles throughout a person's lifetime. To adjust his theory accordingly, he called the initial career choice a maxi-cycle and subsequent career changes mini-cycles.

The multicultural criticisms of Super's theory of career maturity are based on findings that career maturity correlates with socioeconomic status (Smith, 1983). Because career maturity depends on career information and because those in poverty have limited access to career information, the concept of career maturity does not easily translate to this population. Further, the overrepresentation of ethnic minority group members among the poor indicates that the career maturity theory is not applicable to many members of minority cultures either. Research will need to be conducted to determine just what the career developmental stages are for ethnic minorities and those living in poverty. The best approach to such research would be a longitudinal (over time) approach. Most of the research on the career maturity of ethnic minorities has been conducted in the short term.

Life Space

The life space segment of Super's theory involves the various roles people play in their own lives (for instance the roles of parent, child, student, worker, citizen, homemaker, leisurite, and so forth.). The importance or salience an individual places on each of these roles constitutes the individual's life structure (Super et al., 1996). As opposed to the life span segment of Super's theory, the life space segment of the theory is readily adaptable to ethnic minority and other oppressed groups, because it takes into account the individual's perception of his or her world, and because it allows for the differential application of the importance of roles according to the individual's cultural background.

Adapting Career Development Theory for Diverse Clients

As well known and popular as Super's theory was, he was always open to constructive criticism. He genuinely believed that theories are dynamic and that the reason theories are called theories is because they need to be proven. Super was able to adapt a great many facets of his theory to incorporate the lifestyles of groups who were not as privileged as those representing his original research subject pool. Late in his career, Super added what he termed the "archway model" to his theory, wherein he integrated socioeconomic, environmental, and individual factors, which interact and contribute to the career development process (Murray et al., 2002; Super, 1990, 1994). Unfortunately, Super stopped short of incorporating the developmental influences of gender, race, sexuality, and ability status on occupational behavior (Leong & Brown, 1995; Leong & Serfica, 2001).

Career Lifeline Exercise

Draw a career lifeline. Take a letter-size sheet of paper and draw a line down the middle of the page. Turn the page horizontally and starting from one year of age, draw a lifeline of your previous paid and unpaid positions and any milestones that helped you to meet the job requirements (for instance, graduated from high school or college). Put an asterisk next to any major decisions you have made along the way. Once the lifeline is drawn, go back to the asterisks and discuss how the decision was made, whom the decision affected, and if there were any cultural influences that bore on your decision making.

John Holland's Career Theory of Personality Types and Environments

Holland (1966, 1985, 1992, 1997) developed one of the most popular career theories in use today that employs personality types and environments. Compared to the complexity of Super's model, Holland's theory is clear and parsimonious. Essentially, Holland outlines six personality types and six work environments. The six environments are

1. *The Realistic Environment:* A work environment that requires physical strength and agility, and includes many outdoor types of careers
2. *The Investigative Environment:* A work environment that requires dealing with ideas and research
3. *The Artistic Environment:* A work environment that requires creativity and independence
4. *The Social Environment:* A work environment that involves helping people with their problems
5. *The Enterprising Environment :* A work environment that involves influencing people
6. *The Conventional Environment:* A work environment that requires attention to detail and organization

The six personality types parallel the environments, and so in Holland's theory, people's personalities can be broken into six types: those who are realistic, investigative, artistic, social, enterprising, and conventional. Holland theorizes that individuals are most drawn to the work environments that best match their personalities. For example people who are drawn to careers in the enterprising environment enjoy using skills of persuasion to influence others in their personal lives. Further, Holland explains that individuals who enter such career fields are congruent.

To support his theory, Holland (1985, 1994) has developed two popular career assessment instruments, the Vocational Preference Inventory (VPI) and the Self-Directed Search (SDS). Each of these generates an occupational code, which is a combination of the six personality/environments. Individuals use the code to search for occupations with the same code. For example, the results of the SDS may yield an occupational code of Social, Artistic, and Enterprising (SAE). The client would then search for occupations that fall under SAE and learn more about those occupations. Holland codes are also used for the Strong Interest Inventory, which is one of the most widely used career assessment instruments to date.

Two major problems with using Holland's theory with groups who are oppressed by society are (1) that the occupations reflect career stereotypes in terms of gender and ethnicity and (2) that the theory fails to address the impact of race, gender, socioeconomic status, sexual orientation, and ability status. The theory assumes that matching personality with environment is sufficient for clients to locate appropriate jobs (Betz & Fitzgerald, 1987; Carter & Swanson, 1990; Fouad, 1993).

Research has shown that diverse groups tend to score higher on occupations that are traditional or stereotypic for their groups. These are occupations where members of oppressed groups can be found in large numbers and where discrimination against them is minimized. Most of these occupations are lower in prestige and income than occupations populated by white men. For example, women typically score higher on the Social and Conventional codes, African Americans score high on Social, Enterprising, and Conventional codes, and less acculturated Asian Americans score high on Realistic and Investigative codes. Career counselors attempt to assist clients by broadening their ideas about suitable careers. With Holland's theory, rather than generating fresh career ideas for clients to consider, the same traditional fields emerge as possibilities.

In response to the criticism that his theory neglects cultural issues such as race, gender, socioeconomic status, sexual orientation, and ability status, Holland (1997) said that he does not need to address these issues because they are reflected in people's personalities, which are determined by taking the VPI or SDS. In fact, recent studies that have employed Holland's interest inventories, as well as studies that investigate the validity of his theory, have revealed that the theory does, in fact represent the interests of African Americans, Mexican Americans, Asian Americans, Native Americans, and European Americans (Day, Rounds & Swaney, 1998; Sharf, 2002). However, more study is needed before definitive conclusions can be reached. The problem for multicultural clients is not whether or not Holland's inventories measure diverse populations correctly. Rather, the problem is whether or not the messages this theory's results send to the client are appropriate. Even though a theory represents the reality of the society, it does not mean that reality is what is desired. The failure of Holland's theory to recognize the impact that continued oppression may have upon one's ability to pursue a career is a major flaw in the theory and one that will need to be addressed to use this theory with diverse populations (Leong, 1995).

Adapting Holland's Theory for Diverse Clients

The blind spot of Holland's theory is that although Holland's theory seems to adequately predict career choice for ethnic minority groups, it fails to offer a sufficiently wide range of career opportunities for people from minority groups. The multicultural competencies recommend that counselors consider both how sociopolitical influences and pervasive institutional oppression impact individuals. With that in mind, Holland's theory could be adapted to explore how the socialization process discourages women, ethnic minorities, gays, lesbians, bisexuals, and people with disabilities to pursue certain careers. Strategies also need to be developed that separate the skills involved in certain careers from the stereotypical images of these careers Holland's theory often espouses. For example, spatial relations abilities are used in all kinds of occupations, from architecture to window dressing to book design. Helping children develop these abilities regardless of gender will pave the way for plenty of skilled spatial relations workers to enter the workforce, but if we continue to think of such skills as "male" skills, as Holland's theory seems to indicate, we have already lost half the potential workers possessing these skills. The following story from an elementary school counselor, illustrates the importance of overcoming occupational stereotyping.

I was taking a course in techniques of career counseling, and one evening we discussed different strategies to overcome occupational stereotypes. I decided to do something different with my career day in the elementary school where I work. I contacted different professional organizations and told them I wanted a speaker who would be considered nontraditional for the field. For example, I called the fire fighters union and told them that I needed a female speaker. I got some really positive reactions from most of the people I contacted. I was able to find several people who were working in nontraditional fields (a male nurse, a woman carpenter, a male secretary, a female pilot). We played a game with the children on career day. Each child had a set of cards with the career names written on them, and the children put their own names on the backs of the cards. Our visitors introduced themselves and only gave brief clues as to what their professions were. The children then went to the tables where the visitors sat and would give each visitor the career card they thought represented that person's career. The child who got the most careers correct won a prize. After the prize was given, we talked as a class a little about why the children placed the cards where they did. It was a very enlightening experience in debunking occupational stereotypes.

The Holland Code

In his Self-Directed Search, Holland (1994) suggests that individuals recall their occupational daydreams. This is an excellent (though not scientific) method for quickly assessing your personal Holland Code.

1. On a separate sheet of paper list ten occupations that you have ever considered from your childhood to your present age.

2. After you have listed these ten occupations prioritize them from 1 (your most favorite) to 10 (the least favorite of the ten).

3. Now try to identify the Holland Code that best matches each of the ten occupations you listed, and place the first letter of the code next to that occupation. Tally up the number of R's, I's, A's, and so on. The three letters with the most numbers will be your Holland Code. If you have a tie for any of the letters, that is okay, but list both letters.

4. Circle the letters of your Holland Code in the figure. Are the letters next to each other or opposite one another? The closer they are to one another, the more choices you will find. Go to O*Net's interest categories (http://online.onetcenter .org/find/descriptor/browse/Interests/#cur). You should be able to locate careers with all three letters regardless of the order of the letters.

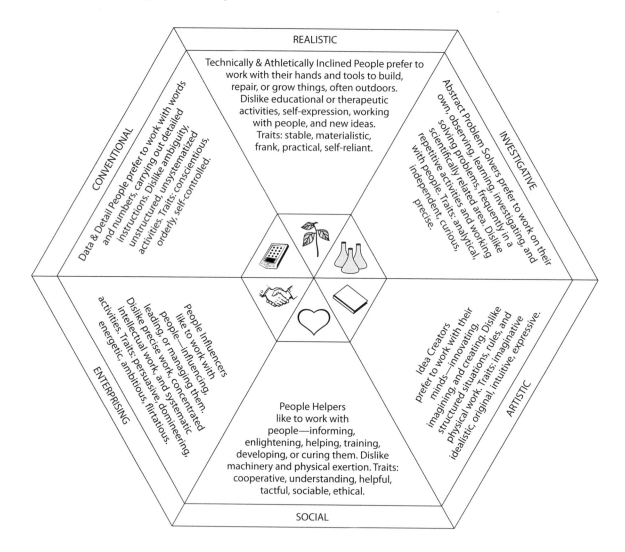

John Krumboltz's Social Learning Theory of Career Development

The social learning theory of career development is typically associated with the work of John Krumboltz (1979). Following the lead of Albert Bandura (1986), Krumboltz developed a theory based on how learning experiences influence career decision making and development. Krumboltz's social learning theory of career counseling purports that people tend to choose careers based on their personal and vicarious learning experiences. According to Krumboltz, one way that learning occurs is through instrumental (reward and punishment) learning. For instance, when individuals are rewarded for a particular behavior, they are inclined to repeat that behavior. If individuals are punished for a particular behavior, they will most likely stop that behavior. Another way that learning occurs is through associative learning, through observation or through conditioning. For example, a girl may observe a woman pediatrician and decide that being a pediatrician is an acceptable occupation for a woman, or a boy who is repeatedly encouraged to build model airplanes may be conditioned to believe that aeronautics is an acceptable occupation for a man. Instrumental learning and associative learning can also have consequences related to race or culture. For instance, if an individual from an ethnic minority group is punished as a child for asking too many questions about a "white" career option, or if the child observes or is repeatedly reminded that a particular profession discriminates against people from his or her cultural group, that individual will likely not pursue a career in that profession.

In 1996, Mitchell & Krumboltz outlined four factors influencing career paths:

- Genetic endowment (one's physical self and one's innate abilities and talents),
- Environmental conditions and events (factors beyond one's control, such as societal changes, acts of nature, and technological advances)
- Learning experiences (instrumental learning and associative learning)
- Task approach skills

When an individual's genetic endowment, environmental conditions, and learning experiences interact, the result is the individual's task approach skills (literally, how the individual approaches performing tasks). In other words, people approach tasks such as career decision making by using their natural abilities, their ability to cope with the world around them, and their observations about themselves and the world.

Putting the above concepts into a career counseling context, Krumboltz (1996) describes how people make their career decisions and provides strategies for helping them with these career choices. According to Krumboltz, people choose occupations that either

1. entail tasks they have succeeded in doing in the past,
2. are valued by significant people in their lives, or
3. they have observed in practice via a role model.

In his most recent writings with others (Mitchell et al., 1999), Krumboltz has added "planned happenstance" to his theory, encouraging clients to prepare for the unexpected (such as encountering discrimination), which may require them to regroup.

There is not much multicultural criticism of Krumboltz's learning theory of career counseling. In fact, most research appears to support the theory. This acceptance is most likely due to the fact that the theory allows for the influence not only of culture, but also of environmental factors outside the control of the client. In addition, there is support for Krumboltz's theory regarding the use of career role models with ethnic minority children. Care must be taken, however, regarding the choice of role models. Children tend to learn best from role models who are closer to their own age and background, rather than from more established, more successful older persons. As a result, the practice of using high school and college students as role models with middle school students will be more successful than pairing middle school students with professional role models who are their parents' age.

RECENT INCLUSIVE THEORIES

As discussed, each of the above four career counseling theories (except Krumboltz's theory) has its own shortcomings regarding multicultural inclusiveness. The two theories discussed below, Gottfredson's developmental model for counseling and social cognitive career theory, manage to avoid such shortcomings.

Linda Gottfredson's Developmental Model for Counseling

Linda Gottfredson (1981) proposed a developmental model for career counseling that helped fill some of the gaps left by Super's theory. Specifically, Gottfredson speaks to gender issues, social class, and motivation that apply across cultures. Expanding upon Super's stages of career development model, Gottfredson's model points out that during early childhood children learn about gender differences; in late childhood, children develop an understanding of social class and prestige; and in adolescence, children gain self-awareness and develop perceptions of others. All of these factors impact the career development stages outlined by Super.

Gottfredson speaks to women and ethnic minorities via her concepts of circumscription and compromise. According to Gottfredson, circumscription involves the narrowing of career choices based on gender in early childhood, and narrowing those choices based on prestige in middle childhood and early adolescence. In other words, children start to eliminate careers they believe are inappropriate for their gender when they are under the age of nine, and they start to eliminate those without prestige after the age of nine. This thinking can be extended to ethnic minority and other oppressed groups. They tend to eliminate careers that seem inappropriate for their cultural group fairly early in their lives.

Compromise involves children changing their career choices as they become more realistic about attaining their careers. In other words, they will let go of choices that seem to be beyond their reach (people like them don't do that kind of work) or that take more effort than they are willing to expend. Gottfredson (2005) states, "compromise is the process by which they [children] begin to relinquish their most preferred alternatives for less compatible but more accessible ones" (p. 82). When compromising, children will sacrifice prestige before they sacrifice a "gender-appropriate" career.

As far as women are concerned, Gottfredson's circumscription and compromise theories both clearly demonstrate how career choices are influenced by gender. As far as ethnic minority groups are concerned, Gottfredson's compromise theory also explains how social class and ethnicity influence career decision making. The idea that people choose careers based on their social accessibility is especially relevant for ethnic minority groups. If one chooses a career that is foreign and unacceptable to the community, one runs the risk of alienating everyone in the community, perhaps making it a career that will take more effort than it is worth.

While there has been research to support the circumscription concept (Henderson, Hesketh, & Tuffin, 1988; Helwig, 1998, 2000), there hasn't been similar support for the compromise concept. In fact, researchers have found that individuals will sacrifice gender-appropriateness for prestige (Hesketh, Durant & Pryor, 1990; Hesketh, Elmslie & Kaldor, 1990), a finding that unfortunately calls the usefulness of Gottfried's theory in terms of women and ethnic minorities into question. However, Lapan, Loehr-Lapan, and Tupper (1993) have designed a promising method for measuring compromise in middle schoolers (Gottfredson & Lapan, 1997; Scharf, 2002).

Social Cognitive Career Theory

A promising new career theory for multicultural career counseling is Social Cognitive Career Theory (SCCT) (Brown & Lent, 1996; Lent, Brown & Hackett, 1994, 1996). Philosophically, it combines the theories of Bandura (1986), Krumboltz (1979), and Hackett and Betz (1981). Although SCCT is similar to Krumboltz's social learning career theory, Lent and colleages (1996) make a distinction between the theories, stating that SCCT focuses more on cognitive processes than social learning career theory's focus on behavior and the interrelationships between personal characteristics, environment, and behavior. Lent's (2005) description of the theory is "SCCT highlights people's capacity to direct their own vocational behavior (human agency) . . . yet it also acknowledges the many personal and environmental influences (such as sociostructural barriers and supports, culture, disability status) that serve to strengthen, weaken, or, in some cases, even override human agency in career development" (p. 102).

There are three factors that drive the SCCT model: self-efficacy, outcome expectations, and personal goals.

Self-efficacy is a term originated by Bandura and refers to a person's belief in his or her own ability to perform a particular task. When asked how confident she would feel about performing an oil change on her car, Ann replies "extremely confident." This indicates that Ann has a strong belief in her ability to do that task or high self-efficacy regarding the task.

Outcome expectations occur when an individual predicts the outcome of an event or interaction; for example, "If I don't graduate in May, then I'll never get a job" or "If I pass the Bar exam, I will have my pick of law firms to work for."

Goals refer to the individual's plans to accomplish certain tasks within a given amount of time—"I will finish my doctorate in three years."

In the SCCT, race/ethnicity, gender, and contextual variables (such as culture and family) as well as learning experience influence self-efficacy and outcome expectations. For instance: CJ is a nineteen-year-old, third generation, Cuban American, middle-class male who has been playing baseball since he was four years old. He has made his college baseball team but has dreams of playing for the major leagues. CJ's parents are proud of his athletic accomplishments and that he is following a family tradition of excellent baseball players—he has an uncle who played in the minor leagues for ten years (FAMILIAL AND CULTURAL SUPPORT). His high batting average and his ability to steal bases (EXPERIENCE) have contributed to his confidence (SELF-EFFICACY). CJ practices longer and harder than others on the team and believes that if he does so, when the major league scouts come to watch his team he will be noticed (OUTCOME EXPECTATION).

The greatest criticism of SCCT comes from those who doubt the usefulness of the concept of self-efficacy with ethnic minority populations. Brown and Lent (1996) point out that self-efficacy for ethnic minorities is influenced by both positive and negative feedback. While an individual may receive positive feedback regarding his or her achievements from European Americans, those same accomplishments may be disparaged by family and friends. These contradictions can lower the individual's self-efficacy and reduce the individual's willingness to pursue careers related to that activity.

SCCT is a complex theory, and while it has yet to be supported for use with multicultural populations, there is great potential for its use with culturally different populations. Swanson and Fouad (1999) point out that the strengths of using this model with multicultural groups are that

(a) the model includes provisions that help counselors identify whether or not clients have made prematurely limited or foreclosed career decisions because of erroneous perceptions of their abilities (e.g. girls can't do math, African Americans can't do science, Asian Americans can't do people);
(b) the model provides an avenue for exploring the barriers clients perceive, barriers that make them eliminate career choices prematurely; and
(c) the model allows for restructuring the client's erroneous beliefs.

Hackett and Byers (1996) point out specific strategies for using SCCT with African American women, particularly with regard to self-efficacy. These ideas are most likely applicable to other oppressed groups. For example, Hackett and Byers recommend that for vicarious learning experience, role models should not only be similar to the client in race and cultural background, but also in age and social background. Counselors can help clients to recognize when the feedback they are given is racially motivated and help them to develop "strong efficacy for coping with racism" (p. 7).

CAREER COUNSELING PROCESS MODELS FOR MULTICULTURAL GROUPS

Three models that are specifically applicable to career counseling with ethnic minority and other oppressed populations will be discussed here. All three of these models are practical models, not philosophically based theories. In other words, contrary to the theories described throughout this chapter, these models focus directly on the counseling process. The three multiculturally focused career models are Leong and Hartung's Integrative Sequential Conceptual Framework for Career Counseling, Fouad and Bingham's (1995) Culturally Appropriate Career Counseling Model (CACCM); and Gold, Rotter, and Evans' (2002) Out of the Box (OTB) model for counseling in the twenty-first century.

Leong and Hartung's Integrative Sequential Conceptual Framework for Career Counseling

Leong and Hartung's (1995) model describes five stages of the career counseling process; stage one occurs prior to the client entering counseling. During stage one, the client recognizes that she or he has career problems and realizes that he or she can benefit from seeing a career counseling specialist. In stage two, the client seeks help for the problem (Leong & Hartung, 1997). To accommodate this stage, it is important that the career agency have staff who are receptive to diverse clienteles, which entails among other things providing bilingual counselors. In stage three, the client's counseling issues are assessed in five dimensions—cultural identity, cultural view of the problem, cultural environmental influences, cultural barriers to counseling, and cultural planning (Swanson & Fouad, 1999). In stage four, the counselor implements the intervention, which may include career assessment. Lastly, in the fifth stage, the client implements his or her career plan. This model assumes that culture will be woven into the counseling throughout the counseling process.

Fouad and Bingham's Culturally Appropriate Career Counseling Model (CACCM)

The CACCM model involves seven steps, beginning with step one, relationship building that is sensitive to the client's culture and counseling expectations. The second step is to assess the client's problem and decide whether the problem is cognitive, social/emotional, behavioral, environmental, and/or external. Step three determines the cultural factors affecting the career problem, using a concentric circle diagram with the client's unique individual qualities at the core of the diagram and circles for gender, family, racial ethnic group, and the dominant majority emanating from the core. Each one of these circles impacts clients differently, depending on clients' career issues or life circumstances (Swanson & Fouad, 1999). Also these factors may interact and affect career choices. In step four, the counselor and client set culturally appropriate goals and culturally sensitive interventions. Steps five and six involve assisting the client in decision making. Finally, in step seven the client executes the plan, and the counselor follows up on client progress.

Gold, Rotter, and Evans' Out of the Box (OTB) Model

Gold, Rotter, and Evans (2002) also advance a process approach called the Out of the Box (OTB) model. They contend that career counseling cannot be done effectively without viewing the client in the context of his or her family and culture. The OTB model challenges counselors who specialize in career counseling, family counseling, and multicultural counseling to develop expertise in all these areas so that they are able to address clients in their entirety. Although Fouad and Bingham (1995) emphasize that counselors need to be culturally competent to implement their model, gaining cultural competence is not one of the steps in the process the authors outlines. Rather, in the OTB model, counselors assess their cultural attitudes and behaviors throughout the counseling relationship.

The counselor and client explore various issues to determine the most salient one for the client at that point in time—that most salient issue is referred to as the client's lifestyle focal point. The lifestyle focal point may be career, family, culture, or any combination of the three. In OTB, the counselor should be able to serve the client's needs, no matter which of these issues or combinations thereof the focal point turns out to be. The counselor then proceeds to work with the client while exploring the following questions:

1. How well do I understand the client's worldview?
    (a) Counselors must assess client problem from multiple perspectives, giving each factor (e.g. abilities, interests, family, culture, gender, income, education, traditions) equal attention.

(b) Counselors need to listen for client priorities with an open mind and resist the temptation to retreat back into the box.

(c) As a result of a and b above, the counselor becomes aware of the client's present lifestyle focal point.

2. How are my own cultural values and biases affecting my approach to this client?

(a) Counselors must realize that the same factors that affect the lifestyle of the client influence their own lifestyle, if perhaps to a different degree or in a different manner.

(b) Counselors should be intimately familiar with their own worldviews, values, and biases, and be aware of how those views could affect the client.

3. Are the interventions I use helpful to my client?

(a) Given the client's lifestyle focal point, the counselor must develop interventions that reflect client need.

(b) The counselor needs to easily move into the sphere of counseling that best fits client needs (family counselors may focus on career issues; career counselors may focus on family issues, and so forth).

(c) The counselor's preferences for working on family, multicultural, or career issues are subordinated by client priorities.

What Is Your Lifestyle Focal Point Exercise

Assume that you are on the brink of making a career or job change. Your lifestyle focal point would be the area of your life that may have had the most influence on your reason for changing careers or positions at this time. To help you identify your lifestyle focal point:

1. List your strengths (may or may not include work related skills)

_____

_____

2. List your weaknesses

_____

_____

3. List your interests/careers (even those other than your own) and leisure activities.

_____

_____

4. List important family facts in your life (spouse/significant other, children, extended family).

_____

_____

5. List cultural factors that are important in your life (gender, ability factors, religion, traditions, language, socioeconomic status, etc.).

_____

_____

When you have completed all five lists, go back and circle ten of the most important factors to you. Then narrow that list down to three of the most important factors to you. The three factors you choose will indicate where your lifestyle focal point will be. If it seems that counseling really needs to be about choosing a new job or career—your focal point is career related. But if family issues turn out to be your major concern, you career issues can wait on hold until you settle problems within the family.

FINAL THOUGHTS ABOUT CAREER COUNSELING THEORIES

Most of the traditional theories can be used with diverse populations as long as counselors are aware that race, ethnicity, gender, sexual orientation, disability, and socioeconomic class must be accounted for. Counselors should challenge those theories that perpetuate occupational stereotypes, such as Holland's theory, by assigning activities that will promote appropriate career alternatives in non-stereotypic occupations. Finally, counselors may want to explore the more inclusive theories or those that are intentionally designed for culturally diverse groups.

Career theories are the maps we use to help clients find their preferred lifestyle. Just as all good map makers know, maps must be updated and changed to reflect population growth and diverse travel needs of map users. Using culturally appropriate applications of career theories, counselors can help all their clients to map out a road in life where they can make decisions effectively, adapt smoothly to a new career or position, and enjoy a fuller, more satisfying lifestyle. We are still searching for the perfect career theory that will fit everyone. Until that is accomplished, we are able to identify the weaknesses of existing theories and adjust them so that they are more comprehensive.

REVIEW/REFLECTION QUESTIONS

Brandi is a twenty-five-year old European American lesbian who has recently graduated from college and is at a stage in her identity development where she is immersed in the lesbian community. She has come out of the closet at work and makes frequent references to her sexual orientation during casual conversations with colleagues and during professional meetings. It seems to Brandi that since she has come out her relationships with her boss and colleagues have been strained. Everyone seems to have kept her at arms' distance and have pretty much isolated her. Brandi has become very disenchanted with her job and comes to you for help finding a new job.

(a) What theory seems to be the best fit for Brandi and her career counseling needs?
(b) Which theory seems to be the least appropriate and explain why?

(c) In the OTB model, counselors are encouraged to explore their attitudes and biases towards their clients. What are your attitudes and biases toward lesbians and how will these affect your work with Brandi?

(d) Using the the theory you chose in a above, outline the steps you would take regarding Brandi's career issue.

REFERENCES

Bandura, A. (1986). *Social foundations of thought and action: A social-cognitive theory.* Upper Saddle River, NJ: Prentice Hall.

Betz, N. E., & Fitzgerald, L. F. (1987). *The career psychology of women.* Orlando, FL: Academic Press.

Bolles, R. N. (2006). *What color is your parachute?* Berkeley, CA: Ten Speed Press.

Brown, S. D., & Lent, R. W. (1996). A social cognitive framework for career choice counseling. *The Career Development Quarterly, 44,* 211–223.

Carter, R. T., & Swanson, J. L. (1990). *Minorities in higher education: Tenth annual status report.* Washington, DC: American Council on Education.

Cass, V. C. (1979). Homosexual identity formation: A theoretical model. *Journal of Homosexuality, 7,* 219–235.

Day, S. X., Rounds, J., & Swaney, K. (1998). The structure of vocational interest for diverse racial-ethnic groups. *Psychological Science, 9,* 40–44.

Dillard, J. M., & Perrin, D. W. (1980). Puerto Rican, Black, and Anglo adolescents' career aspirations, expectations, and maturity. *Vocational Guidance Quarterly, 28,* 313–321.

Fouad, N. A. (1993). Cross-cultural vocational assessment. *The Career Development Quarterly, 42,* 4–13.

Fouad, N. A., & Bingham, R. (1995). Career counseling with racial/ethnic minorities. In W. B. Walsh & S. H. Osipow (Eds.), *Handbook of vocational psychology* (2nd ed.; pp. 331–366). Hillscale, NJ: Lawrence Erlbaum.

Gold, J. G., Rotter, J. C., & Evans, K. M. (2002). Out of the box: A model for counseling in the twenty-first century. In K. M. Evans, J. C. Rotter & J. G. Gold (Eds.), *Synthesizing family, career, and culture: A model for counseling in the twenty-first century* (pp. 19–33). Alexandria, VA: American Counseling Association.

Gottfredson, L (2005). Applying Gottfredson's theory of circumscription and compromise in career guidance and counseling. In S. D. Brown & R. W. Lent (Eds.). *Career development and counseling: Putting theory and research to work* (pp. 71–100). Hoboken, NJ: John Wiley & Sons, Inc

Gottfredson, L. S. (1981). Circumscription and compromise: A developmental theory of occupational aspirations. *Journal of Counseling Psychology, 28,* 545–579.

Gottfredson, L. S. (1986). Special groups and the beneficial use of vocational interest inventories. In W. B. Walsh & S. H. Osipow (Eds.) *Advances in vocational psychology, Vol. 1: The assessment of interests* (pp. 127–198). Hillsdale, NJ: Lawrence Erlbaum Associates, Inc, 1986.

Gottfredson, L. S., & Lapan, R. T. (1997). Assessing gender-based circumscription of occupational aspirations, *Journal of Career Assessment, 5,* 419–441.

Hackett, G., & Betz, N. E. (1981) A self-efficacy approach to the career development of women. *Journal of Vocational Behavior, 18,* 326–339.

Hackett, G., & Byars, A. (1996). Social cognitive theory and the career development of African American women. *The Career Development Quarterly, 44,* 322–340.

Hartung, P. J., Vandiver, B. J., Leong, F. T. L., Pope, M., Niles, S. G., & Farrow, B. (1998). Appraising cultural identity in career development assessment and counseling. *Career Development Quarterly, 46,* 276–293.

Helwig, A. A. (1998). Gender-role stereotyping: Testing theory with a longitudinal sample. *Sex Roles, 38,* 403–423.

Helwig, A. A. (2001). A test of Gottfredson's theory using a ten-year longitudinal study, *Journal of Career Development, 28,* 77–95.

Henderson, S., Hesketh, B., & Tuffin, A. (1988). A test of Gottfredson's theory of circumscription. *Journal of Vocational Behavior, 32,* 37–48.

Herr, E. L., Cramer, S. H., & Niles, S. G. (2004). *Career guidance and counseling through the lifespan: Systematic approaches.* Boston: Pearson Education, Inc.

Hesketh, B., Durant, C., & Pryor, R. (1990). Career compromise: A test of Gottfredson's (1981) theory using a policy-capturing procedure. *Journal of Vocational Behavior, 36,* 97–108.

Hesketh, B., Elmslie, S., & Kaldor, W. (1990). Career compromise: An alternative account to Gottfredson's theory. *Journal of Counseling Psychology, 37,* 40–56.

Holland, J. L. (1966) *The psychology of vocational choice.* Waltham, MA: Blaisdell.

Holland, J. L. (1985). *Making vocational choices: A theory of vocational personalities and work environments* (2nd ed.). Upper Saddle River, NJ: Prentice Hall.

Holland, J. L. (1992). *Making vocational choices* (2nd ed.) Odessa, FL: Psychological Assessment Resources.

Holland, J. L. (1997). *Making vocational choice: A theory of vocational personalities and work environments* (3rd ed.). Odessa, FL: Psychological Assessment Resources.

Krumboltz, J. D. (1979). A social learning theory of career decision-making. In A. M. Mitchell, G.B. Jones & J. D. Krumboltz (Eds.) *Social Learning and career decision making* (pp. 19–49). Cranston, RI: Carroll Press.

Krumboltz, J. D. (1996). A learning theory of career counseling. In M. L. Savickas & W. B. Walsh (Eds.), *Handbook of career counseling theory and practice* (pp. 55–80). Paulo Alto, CA: Davies-Black.

Lapan, R. T. Loehr-Lapan, S. J., & Tupper, T. W. (1993). *Tech-prep careers workbook: Counselor's manual.* Columbia Department of Educational and Counseling Psychology, University of Missouri-Columbia.

Lent, R. W. (2005). A Social Cognitive View of Career Development and Counseling. In. S. D. Brown & R. W. Lent (Eds.). *Career development and counseling: Putting theory and research to work* (pp. 101–127). Hoboken, NJ: John Wiley & Sons, Inc.

Lent, R. W., Brown, S. D., & Hackett, G. (1994). Toward a unifying social cognitive theory of career and academic interests, choice, and performance. *Journal of Vocational Behavior, 45,* 79–122.

Lent, R. W., Brown, S. D., & Hackett, G. (1996). Career development from a social cognitive perspective. In D. Brown, L. Brooks & Associates (Eds.), *Career choice and development* (4th ed.; pp. 255–311). San Francisco, CA: Jossey-Bass.

Leong, F. T. L. (1995). *Career development and vocational behavior of racial and ethnic minorities.* Hillsdale, NJ, England: Lawrence Erlbaum Associates, Inc.

Leong, F. T. L., & Brown, M. T. (1995). Theoretical issues in cross-cultural career development: Cultural validity and cultural specificity. In W. B. Walsh & S. H. Osipow (Eds.). *Handbook of vocational psychology: Theory, research, and practice* (2nd ed.) (pp. 143–180). Hillsdale, NJ: Lawrence Erlbaum Associates, Inc.

Leong, F. T. L., & Hartung, P. J. (1997). Career assessment with culturally different clients: Proposing an integrative-sequential conceptual framework for cross-cultural career counseling research and practice. *Journal of Career Assessment, 5,* 183–201.

Leong, F. T. L., & Serafica, F. C. (2001). Cross-cultural perspective on Super's career development theory: Career maturity and cultural accommodation. In F. T. Leong & A. Barak, *Contemporary models in vocational psychology: A volume in honor of Samuel H. Osipow* (pp. 167–205). Mahwah, NJ, US: Lawrence Erlbaum Associates, Publishers.

McNamara, K., & Rickard, K. M. (1989). Feminist identity development: Implications for feminist therapy with women. *Journal of Counseling & Development, 68,* pp. 184–189.

Mitchell, L. K., Levin, A. S., & Krumboltz, J. D. (1999). Planned happenstance: Constructing unexpected career opportunities. *Journal of Counseling and Development, 77,* 115–124.

Mitchell, L. K., & Krumboltz, J. D. (1996). Krumboltz's theory of career choice and counseling. In D. Brown, L. Brooks & Associates (Eds.) *Career choice development* (3rd ed.; pp. 233–380). San Francisco, CA: Jossey-Bass.

Murray, P., Williamson, L., Boudrot, K., Reents, E., Roberts, T., & Evans, K. M. (2002). Synthesizing career and family theories: Relevant issues. In K. M. Evans, J. C. Rotter & J. G. Gold (Eds.), *Synthesizing family, career, and culture: A model for counseling in the twenty-first century* (pp. 35–60). Alexandria, VA: American Counseling Association.

Neville, H. A., Gysbers, N. C., Heppner, M. J., & Johnston, J. (1998). Empowering life choices: Career counseling in cultural contexts. In N. C. Gysbers, M. J. Heppner & J. Johnston, *Career counseling: Process, issues, and techniques.* Boston: Allyn & Bacon.

Niles, S. G., & Harris-Bowlsbey, J. (2005). *Career development interventions in the 21st Century* (2nd ed.). Upper Saddle River, NJ: Pearson Merrill Prentice Hall.

Parham, T. A., & Helms, J. E. (1985). Relation of racial identity attitudes to self-actualization and affective states of Black students. *Journal of Counseling Psychology, 32,* 431–440.

Parsons, F. (1909). *Choosing a vocation.* Garrett Park, MD: Gerrett Park Press.

Prince, J. P., Uemura, A. K., Chao, C. S., & Gonzales, G. M. (1991). Using career interest inventories with multicultural clients. *Career Planning and Adults Development Journal, 45*–50.

Sharf, R. F. (2002). *Applying career development theory to counseling.* Pacific Grove, CA: Wadsworth Group.

Smith, E. J. (1983) Issues in racial minorities career behavior. In W. B. Walsh & S. H. Osipow (Eds.), *Handbook of vocational psychology, Volume 1, Foundations.* Hillsdale, NJ: Lawrence Erlbaum.

Super, D. E. (1957). *The psychology of careers.* New York: Harper & Row.

Super, D. E. (1990). A life-span, life-space approach to career development. In D. Brown, L. Brooks & Associates (Eds.), *Career choice and development: Applying contemporary theories to practice* (2nd ed., pp. 197–261). San Francisco, CA: Jossey-Bass.

Super, D. E. (1994). A life-span, life-space perspective on convergence. In M. L. Savickas & R. W. Lent (Eds.), *Convergence in career development theories* (pp. 63–74). Palo Alto, CA: Consulting Psychologists Press.

Super, D. E., Osborne, W. L., Walsh, D. J., Brown, S. D., & Niles, S. G. (1992). Developmental assessment and counseling: The C-DAC model, *Journal of Counseling and Development, 71,* 74–80.

Super, D. E., Savickas, M. L., & Super, C. M., (1996). The life-span, life-space approach to careers. In D. Brown, L. Brooks, & Associates (Eds.), *Career choice and development* (3rd ed., pp. 121–178). San Francisco: Jossey-Bass.

Swanson, J. L., & Fouad, N. A. (1999). *Career theory and practice: Learning through case studies.* Thousand Oaks, CA: Sage Publications, Inc.

CHAPTER 6
Cultural Competence in Testing

Malachi is a seventeen-year-old, African American high school senior who has come to counseling to discuss his life after high school. He has not made any decisions about what he wants to do, and every time he has seen his high school counselor in the past, he has changed his mind about his goals. Malachi is an average student who has received mainly Bs and Cs in his classes. He has taken enough of the right courses, and he has gotten adequate grades to enter the local community college or a two-year technical college. However, his grades indicate that he would not be competitive at a four-year college or university. His counselor, Jim (a white male), assumes that part of his task is to help Malachi assess his career aspirations, perhaps by administering career tests. Because he has received some training in multicultural counseling, Jim is aware that there are issues related to testing for members of diverse groups. Therefore, he is hesitant about traditional testing instruments. Malachi is his first African American student, and Jim wants to be certain that he does what is best for Malachi. Jim decides that he needs more direction and guidance to work with Malachi, so he asks a colleague, who is well trained in multicultural career counseling, to supervise his work with this client.

Jim is making a culturally sensitive and ethical decision. He realizes that he lacks the expertise to serve his client in the most effective manner possible, and he is seeking assistance so that he will learn more and be better prepared to handle clients like Malachi in the future. For Jim to be culturally competent in his work with Malachi, he not only will have to tap into his knowledge about cultural differences, but he will also need to learn to evaluate and interpret tests so that Malachi will reap the largest possible benefits from them. Jim may also need to learn alternative means of assessment, which may be more appropriate for the various members of his culturally diverse clientele than standard means of assessment.

Testing has been the cornerstone of career counseling since its inception (Gainor, 2000). In fact, skills in testing and in providing career information are the areas of expertise that most distinguish career counselors from other counseling specialists. Traditionally, career assessment includes tests of ability and/or aptitude, along with interest, value, and personality inventories. Career counselors administer tests to help clients access information about themselves that they would otherwise be unable to do in an expedient manner. The information clients learn about themselves includes their needs, their values, their interests, their abilities, and their career development progress (Niles & Bowlesby, 2005). The results of the tests are interpreted either to diagnose client problematic areas or to assist clients with subsequent decision making (Subich, 1996). Therefore, counselors take testing courses that typically focus on the technical qualities and the diagnostic nature of the tests. This narrow focus can result in administering tests without taking into account a holistic view of a client and may result in the ineffective or unethical evaluation and application of test results. The misuse of tests has been common in the past and has led to testing and career counseling being referred to as "three sessions and a cloud of dust," meaning that the three-session practice, which included testing, left clients more confused than helped. Today, standards and ethical codes regarding test usage are well established.

While the Association for Assessment in Counseling and Education (AACE) has published specific standards for the use of tests with multicultural populations, the selection and use of standardized tests with diverse populations requires specialized skills that are not explicitly addressed in any of the standards (AACE, 2003). According to Ridley, Li, and Hill (1998), little guidance has been given to counselors regarding multicultural assessment. "Clinicians are left to their own judgment as to what data to collect, how the data are to be collected, and how to organize and evaluate data" (p. 847). Constantine (1998) eloquently lists the potential pitfalls of testing diverse populations; these include "inappropriate test content, examiner and language bias, inappropriate standardization samples, inequitable social consequences, unclear concept equivalence (i.e. whether a particular psychological construct has equivalent or similar meanings within and across various cultural groups), different predictive validity, and differences in test-taking skills" (p. 924).

The concerns of these authors are real and still current. As recently as a decade ago, it was not uncommon for the standardization samples of career tests and inventories to include no people of color. Test developers operated under the culturally encapsulated assumption that all test takers would be similar to the white, European American, middle-class, nondisabled population upon which tests were normed. Because of these assumptions, not only is little known about the career development of many oppressed groups, but also little is known about the applicability of career assessment to diverse populations (Ridley, Li & Hill, 1998). The issue has become even more complicated as a result of the tremendous growth and availability of online career assessments (Chartrand & Walsh, 2001). Because online testing usually generates preconstructed and standard interpretations, they typically do not take into consideration cultural differences and may generate inappropriate interpretations. Without counselor input into these interpretations, clients may be adversely affected by online testing. Combining the competencies of the National Career Development Association (NCDA) and Association for Multicultural Counseling and Development (AMCD) regarding testing is an essential step toward insuring that career assessment testing applies to all groups. Therefore, this chapter will focus on the integration of the NCDA and AMCD competencies (which are outlined in Figure 6.1) by first outlining the types of tests offered, then exploring cultural and environmental factors as they apply to career testing, and finally tying these factors together via a discussion of test interpretation models.

Figure 6.1   NCDA and AMCD competencies

The NCDA competencies career counselors must master are the ability to

1. Assess personal characteristics such as aptitude, achievement, interests, values, and personality traits
2. Assess leisure interests, learning style, life roles, self-concept, career maturity, vocational identity, career indecision, work environment preference (e.g., work satisfaction), and other related lifestyle/development issues
3. Assess conditions of the work environment, such as tasks, expectations, norms, and qualities of the physical and social settings
4. Evaluate and select valid and reliable instruments appropriate to the client's gender, sexual orientation, race, ethnicity, and physical and mental capacities
5. Use computer-delivered assessment measures effectively and appropriately
6. Select assessment techniques appropriate for group administration and those appropriate for individual administration
7. Administer, score, and report findings from career-assessment instruments appropriately
8. Interpret data from assessment instruments and present the results to clients and to others
9. Assist the client and others designated by the client to interpret data from assessment instruments
10. Write an accurate report of assessment results

The AMCD competencies career counselors must master are the ability to

1. interpret assessment results including implications of dominant cultural values affecting assessment/interpretation, the interaction of cultures for those who are bicultural, and the impact of historical institutional oppression
2. discuss information regarding cultural, racial, gender profile of normative group used for validity and reliability on any assessment
3. understand the limitations of translating assessment instruments as well as the importance of using language that includes culturally relevant connotations and idioms
4. [Administer and evaluate] assessment instruments appropriately for clients having limited English skills
5. [Provide] examples for each assessment instrument used, of the limitations of the instrument regarding various groups (p. 28)

Reproduced with permission from NCDA.

TYPES OF CAREER TESTS

In order for counselors to utilize career testing to the greatest advantage of their clients, they must understand the societal influences that create testing bias. Until society changes or a truly culturally fair test is developed, counselors must be mindful of how they select, administer, and interpret the results of potentially biased tests. Career counselors must not only be aware of cultural bias in testing, but also do their homework to be certain that the tests they choose are appropriate for the members of the oppressed groups they will be serving. Without such consideration, counselors risk perpetuating "an oppressive system that denies equal access to occupational opportunity to all" (Gainor, 2000, p. 170). The discussion below outlines issues related to three different types of standardized tests commonly used in career counseling: interest inventories, aptitude and ability tests, and personality tests.

Interest Inventories

Interest inventories are administered to help clients make career decisions by focusing on client interests rather than on existing abilities or financial resources. Counselors usually assign interest inventories to clients to help them expand their ideas about possible careers. This expansion of choices does not always occur naturally among culturally different groups. Due to limited societal options, their perceived interests tend to cluster around a small range of career choice possibilities, and interest inventories tend to confirm that tendency. As a result, ethnic minorities and white women find themselves presented with limited career options (Gainor, 2000). Several studies have been conducted, which are geared toward determining if interest inventories are appropriate to use with ethnic minority groups. Carter and Swanson (1990) state emphatically that the Strong Interest Inventory (SII) is not valid for African Americans, but subsequent research has found that Holland's hexagonal theory, which is part of the SII, is useful with ethnic minority groups (Anderson, Tracey & Rounds, 1997; Day & Rounds 1998; Fouad, Harmon & Borgen, 1997). The problem is that SII is still heavily reliant on a predominantly white reference group, and that small normative group is inappropriately applied to all clients, ethnic minority or otherwise. As with many standardized tests, the Strong was updated and re-normed in 1994. It was the first time in the history of the test that a racial breakdown was obtained for the norm group. Unfortunately, the new normative sample still came up disappointingly short in terms of diversity. Although ethnic minority group members make up over 25 percent of the U.S. population, only one third of the 98 criterion groups in the new SII update included ethnic minority representation, and of those groups only 18 percent featured minority representation of over 10 percent (Kelly, 2003). This caveat is supported by Kelly (2003) who reports in his review that "it is evident that the Strong . . . fails to represent the racial and ethnic diversity of the U.S." (p. 897). The SII manual states that although no real conclusions can be made about the above findings due to the sampling procedure, the SII has begun to address the issue of diversity in their testing samples (Harmon et al., 1994). In addition to including racial minority groups in the occupational samples in the 1994 revision, several minor changes were also made to increase gender fairness. Interestingly, although the gender gap within traditional occupations has narrowed as women continue to move into occupations traditionally reserved for men, there still are enough differences between how women score items on interest inventories to warrant continuation of separate scales for men and women. When the SII was first developed, there was a form for men and a separate form for women. Eventually the two forms were merged but the results for men and women were never combined. In fact recent research on SII items found that there were differences between men and women on 97 items and that these differences were substantial enough to warrant the development of a separate scale that reflected gender differences (Harmon et al., 1994). Similarly, a study on sexual orientation as it pertains to career interests by Chung and Harmon (1994) found that there are measurable patterns of career preferences for gay men that differ from those of straight men. Using the SII (which incorporates the Holland occupational codes) research found that gay men score lower on the Realistic and Investigative occupations and higher on the Artistic and Social occupations. In fact, Croteau and colleagues (2000) suggest that gay men and lesbians tend to choose nontraditional careers more often than heterosexual men and women. Unfortunately, culturally encapsulated counselors often try to discourage their gay and lesbian clients from choosing these nontraditional careers, even though these careers may be the best fit for these clients (Harmon et al., 1994).

The Strong interest inventory manual offers an entire section for use with clients with disabilities, which provides administration and interpretation recommendations (Harmon et al., 1994). This section stresses individual attention to the needs of persons with disabilities, whether that means darkening in the bubbles on the answer sheet for the client or reading the inventory questions aloud to test takers—whatever will improve the client's chances of giving an accurate picture of the client. Further, DeWitt (1994) suggests that the SII may be helpful in (a) evaluating a client's abilities and accommodating the environment to enhance abilities; (b) gaining focus in career planning; (c) reducing stereotypical occupational placements (i.e. stuffing envelopes) and encouraging a wide range of choices; and (d) facilitating re-entry into the workplace. Much of the research on people with disabilities shows their interests do not differ from people without disabilities including the dissimilar interests of men and women. Counselor awareness of the interests of people with disabilities is likely to result in an openness to treating these clients.

Aptitude Tests

The types of tests that have received the most criticism in terms of bias are aptitude tests, particularly intelligence tests that measure cognitive abilities. These tests purport to predict academic and professional performance, yet ethnic minority groups routinely score lower than European Americans on them. The reasons for ethnic differences are difficult to determine, but those differences do exist (Helms, 1992; Neisser et al., 1996).

The fact that people of diverse backgrounds perform differently on cognitive ability tests, as well as on other career assessments has raised questions about the validity of using tests on clients from diverse backgrounds at all. Books, articles, and other literature concerning differential test performance results have proliferated over the years, although in the end most of the conclusions have been contradictory, often contentious, in fact, when it comes to determining the causes of the differences. On the racist side of the coin, one faction supports the contention that culturally different individuals (primarily African Americans) tend to score lower on standardized aptitude tests because they are innately less intelligent than whites (Jensen, 1998). The response from African Americans and others has been to argue that the test differences do not stem from innate intelligence differences, rather from the fact that intelligence tests are inherently biased against those who are culturally different. The most recent flurry of debate regarding this issue occurred with the publication of *The Bell Curve* in 1994. In this book, Herrnstein and Murray (1994) concluded that the difference in IQ scores between racial groups is genetically determined. While psychologists debate the validity of the research and conclusions made by Hernstein and Murray, the bottom line for career counselors is that they should be aware that such research and status quo acceptance of such thinking perpetuates the idea that African Americans, and Latinas and Latinos, are intellectually inferior and often harms the career development and career choices of ethnic minority individuals throughout their lives.

Interestingly, the differences in aptitude scores between ethnic minority and dominant groups is less substantial than the differences within groups (Hartman, McDaniel & Whetzel, 2003). For instance, there are greater differences between low-income and middle-income Latinas and Latinos than there are between Latinos and Latinas, and European Americans. In fact, recent studies show that aptitude tests are as predictive for ethnic minority groups as they are for whites (Betz, 1992). Although these findings may not be cause for celebration, the findings do show that the tests are a reflection of an oppressive society, and that the tests accurately predict how persons who are economically oppressed will fare in that society.

The most well-known aptitude test, the Scholastic Aptitude Test (SAT) is used by colleges and universities to determine admission eligibility. It, too, was reconstructed in 1994 to address the issue of bias. The result of the revision was that scores among women and minorities increased over time (College Board, n.d.). However, according to Freedle (2003), the SAT continues to show ethnic bias. As a result, lower scores received by ethnic minorities (along with the declining use of affirmative action in college admission) have led to a decrease in ethnic minority college enrollment and a subsequent decrease in ethnic minority attainment of professional careers (Freeman, 1997, 1999; Walpole et al., 2005).

Further, the knowledge among ethnic minorities that their group performs consistently lower on aptitude tests may have a significant effect on test performance itself. In other words, knowing the expectations applied to them, members of ethnic minority groups don't expect to perform well on these tests and therefore are subject to stresses that inhibit their testing abilities. Students may perceive some stigma in being a member of an ethnic minority group when it comes to test performance. This in and of itself affects test performance.

Steele and Aronson (1995) have conducted research on test takers to see if an individual's association of race and low aptitude test scores actually influences that individual's test performance. Specifically, Steele and Aronson performed a series of studies on the effect negative stereotypes may have on the test performances of African Americans. The phenomenon they were interested in was "stereotype threat," or the fear that a negative stereotype may be applied to oneself. According to the researchers, "any test that purports to measure intellectual ability might induce stereotype threat in African American students" (p. 404). In one of their studies, Steele and Aronson found that even the mention of race in conjunction with testing resulted in poorer performance of African Americans as compared to whites and blacks in a control group. In this study, 47 undergraduates (6 black males, 18 black females, 11 white males, and 12 white females) were randomly assigned to one of two test conditions—one that required participants to indicate their racial identity and the other that did not require racial identification. All other testing procedures and instruments were identical. Students were asked to complete a very difficult verbal aptitude test and were told not to expect to do well on it. After completing the test, the students completed a questionnaire designed to determine their reactions not just to the tests, but also to the questions on stereotype threat preceding the test. Steele and Aronson found that the African Americans students who were asked to identify themselves racially performed worse than any other test participants—not only the white students, but also the African American students who were not asked to identify their race. As a result of this study and others in the series, Steel and Aronson concluded that "compared to viewing the problem of black underachievement as rooted in something about the group or its societal conditions, this analysis uncovers a social psychological predicament of race, rife in the standardized testing situation that is amenable to change . . ." (p. 819).

Personality Tests

Personality tests are often used in career counseling to help clients gain an understanding of how their personal characteristics fit the requirements of different professions. These tests also show clients how much they might personally have in common with potential colleagues. Personality tests are sometimes administered by potential employers as well, to help employers reduce the risk of hiring unsuitable employees.

The 16PF is a popular personality test, and like other standardized tests, it was also re-normed in 1994. A few major changes to the fifth edition of the 16PF included removing racially-biased, gender-biased, and ability-status biased language from the test, and removing test items that might not be easily translated by those for whom English is a second language. In addition, 16PF added a test of general reasoning ability comparable to an IQ test. Not unlike in other aptitude tests, the authors of the 16PF revision found that race was a factor in the scoring of the reasoning subtest, though gender was not. For example, they found that Asians and whites tend to score higher on the reasoning test than Hispanics, Native Americans, or African Americans.

Types of Tests as Applied to Malachi's Situation

This chapter opened with a vignette centering on Malachi, an African American high school senior who is exploring with his guidance counselor, Jim, whether or not he should enter the local community college, enroll at a technical college, or directly enter the workforce following his graduation. The following continuation of the vignette reveals that Malachi has now added joining the navy as one of his options and illustrates how Malachi's counseling experience is impacted by the pros and cons of the types of tests discussed above when administered to ethnic minority students:

Since Malachi was interested in learning more about how well he might compete with others going to college, as well as those going into the navy for training, Jim suggests that Malachi take two specific aptitude tests—the SAT and the ASVAB (the Armed Services Vocational Aptitude Battery). Jim consults his colleague about her experiences in discussing and interpreting these instruments for African American students. He also does some reading on the pros and cons of these tests regarding African Americans to help with his follow-up talk with Malachi. He learns that aptitude tests tend to be as predictive for African Americans and other minorities as they are for whites. In other words, these tests do predict how well students will perform in the armed services or in colleges that accept their test scores. Jim will also report to Malachi the typical SAT scores earned by other African American students at the high school who were accepted at various colleges and universities. Jim is happy that the senior counselor has kept data on students who graduated and the universities they enrolled in. Jim will share that information with Malachi as well.

Jim's choice to administer the SAT and the ASVAB is appropriate, even though African Americans score lower than whites on these tests. Both tests are required for admission by colleges (SAT) or the military (ASVAB). More importantly, Jim's plan to discuss Malachi's results compared with the average scores for African American graduates from his high school who have been admitted to college will help Malachi develop a realistic evaluation of his chances to be admitted to college or the military training he desires.

CULTURAL AND ENVIRONMENTAL INFLUENCES ON CAREER TESTING

In addition to problems with various types of career tests themselves, cultural and environmental factors also influence the testing experience.

Cultural Influences

A number of authors in the counseling field have reminded counselors that they must be secure in their own cultures before they can work with the cultural issues of clients. Further, Arredondo and colleagues (1996), Flores, Spanierman, and Obasi (2003), Highlen and Sudarsky-Gleiser (1994), and Ridley and colleagues (1998) have indicated that counselors must be willing to explore client cultural background deeply before moving on to the testing stage.

The AMCD, NCDA, and the Association for Assessment in Counseling and Education (AACE) all have highlighted the importance of recognizing cultural differences in career assessment. In its Standards for Multicultural Assessment (a compilation of professional standards this organization put together from five different sources), AACE includes thirteen standards for selection of tests, sixteen standards for administration of the tests, and twenty-one standards for the interpretation of assessment results (NCDA, 1997). Some of the cultural differences among people that may influence their testing results (as well as the counselor's interpretation of these results) include values and beliefs, age, ethnicity, racial identity, gender, language and acculturation, sexual orientation, and ability status. The cultural factors that have received the most attention in the literature are values and beliefs, acculturation, race and ethnicity, language, and gender. However, since the implementation of the Americans with Disabilities Act (ADA), more consideration has been given to the needs of people with disabilities; and the cultural factors that influence the careers of gay men, lesbians, and bisexuals have received more attention recently, due to a great degree to these groups' own efforts to increase sensitivity to their career issues. The following sections outline ways in which values and beliefs, race/ethnicity/sexual orientation/gender, cultural/racial identity, and acculturation/language affect performance and outcomes in career testing.

Values and Beliefs

In collective cultures that value interdependence (such as Latino and Native American cultures), individual tests rarely affect only the test taker. In these cultures, the individual is subordinate to the group. Therefore, when an individual takes a test, the outcome is important to the entire group (LaFramboise et al., 1990). When one does well, this reflects positively on the group, and one's failures reflect negatively on the group. Counselors must keep this in mind when assigning any kind of standardized test to people from collective cultures (Fukuyama & Cox, 1992). While keeping cultural collectiveness in mind, however, counselors must also keep in mind that some individuals from these collective cultures may have adopted the Western and European American values of individuality (Ridley, Li & Hill, 1998).

An intriguing example of how values and beliefs influence career testing is that certain cultural groups typically choose certain occupations in common when taking interest inventories. For example, on the SII, African American males and females score high on social careers, whereas Asian Americans score high on math and science careers. One cannot help but think that the cultural influence is strong, that the values and beliefs individuals cherish manifest themselves via career choice. Meir and Tziner (2001) have pointed out the strong influence culture can have on the career choices of members of a cultural group. They used Hofstede's (1986) classification of cultures to outline the careers that most closely relate to the values of the cultural groups. African Americans, for example tend to have collectivist and communal values that are most readily represented by social occupations. Asian Americans, although also collectivist, tend to avoid ambiguity and uncertainty, a choice that science and math careers tend to reflect.

Race/Ethnicity/Sexual Orientation/Gender

The effect of race and ethnicity on test performance has been perhaps the most hotly debated topic in the field of career counseling. The original impetus for the debate was Jensen's research on intelligence, in which Jensen concluded that African Americans are intellectually inferior to whites (Jensen, 1980). The reverberations of this conclusion can still be felt today. Studies have continued to show that whites and Asians score higher on standardized aptitude tests than Hispanics, who in turn score higher than African Americans (Hartman et al., 2003). However, alternate research espouses that aptitude tests are biased, because items on these tests require information more readily available in white culture (Loehlin, Lindzey & Spuhlerg, 1975). For gay, lesbian, bisexual, and transgender clients, SII results may be affected by heterosexist assumptions on the part of test developers and examiners (Whitcomb, Wettersen & Stolz, 2006). An example is the use of heterosexual norms on the "Infrequent Response" scale of the Strong Interest Inventory. The Infrequent Response Scale was developed by creating items most people would answer a certain way. For example, if most people are asked if they would like to win a million dollars, they would say yes and if someone were to say no, that would be different from the majority of people and would be counted as an infrequent response. One assumption about this kind of response would be that the examinee may not be reading the test but instead may be randomly filling in the test bubbles. When there are enough infrequent responses, the results of the SII are considered invalid. Examinees with enough nontraditional responses (such as teacher for men, construction worker for women) are in danger of having their whole test thrown out. Counselors should be aware that this kind of normative generalization is culturally encapsulated and is found not only in the SII but also on other tests. When career counselors interpret the results of SII for gay, lesbian, bisexual, or transgendered clients, they should be aware that the gender-based occupational scale of the SII should be accompanied by further exploration, because these clients may fit certain occupational roles better than the test results might indicate.

Cultural/Racial Identity

An individual's acceptance of his or her racial or cultural identity may also have an impact on the results of standardized testing. Subich (1996) suggests that simply noting the race of a client is insufficient when interpreting test results—the counselor must address racial identity to "fully appreciate individual differences" (p. 285). According to Gainor (2000), several studies have investigated the relationship between racial identity and career development and have concluded that racial identity is important to explore (Evans and Herr, 1994; Gainor and Lent, 1998). For example, individuals at the Conformity or Dissonance identity stages are more likely to experience internalized racism, which has been found to negatively affect self-efficacy and which may, in turn, result in clients limiting their own career choices on interest inventories (Betz & Hackett, 1981; Highlen & Sudarsky-Gliser, 1994). Clients in the Resistance Stage may be particularly outraged by racism and may refuse to participate in testing at all.

Assessment of a client's cultural/racial identity may be conducted through an interview with the client. Counselors familiar with the models can take educated guesses about the client's attitudes; however, there are several more formal assessment instruments that may be appropriate. For example, Parham and Helms's Racial Identity Attitude Scale has been widely used in research.

Acculturation and Language

Acculturation is the degree to which individuals adopt or conform to cultures different from their own. More often than not, acculturation refers to the degree to which racial and ethnic minority group members adopt the values and lifestyles of the dominant European American culture (Lee & Chuang, 2005; Lee, 1997). It is tempting for counselors to predict how clients from particular cultures will think, behave, or emotionally react to testing. However, an assessment of acculturation needs to be conducted before such predictions may be applied to any specific client. Because ethnic minorities generally function within the dominant culture in their jobs or in the educational arena, they learn to maneuver between two different cultures—their own culture at home and the dominant culture at work or at school. Some individuals are able to separate their experiences and move in and out of the two cultures with ease. These types of people are considered to be highly acculturated because they know how to function in the dominant society without completely abandoning their own culture. Recent immigrants, on the other hand, are less likely to be acculturated and will tend to place major importance on preserving their own culture (Berry, 1980; LeVine & Padilla, 1981). In their research of an acculturation scale, Olmedo and Padilla (1978) found that language was the best predictor of acculturation—the more acculturated people are, the more likely they are to speak English. Assessing a client's level of acculturation is important in test selection and interpretation. The more acculturated a client is, the more helpful standardized tests will be. Conversely, tests are probably not useful at all for clients whose acculturation level is low because clients may lack the fluency in English needed to perform well on the test, tests translated for clients may be suspect, and tests geared toward and normed based on European American culture are not likely to provide clients with accurate information about themselves (Hansen, 1987; Highlen & Sudarsky-Gleiser, 1994).

Another important consideration is that even when tests are translated, words don't always have equal meaning across language, and various nuances of the original test's language may be lost in translation, resulting in skewed test results (Hanson, 1987). The same problem may occur when counselors use interpreters to explain test results to clients. In the AACE standards, test developers are encouraged to assess the validity of translated tests. Test administrators should review that information before deciding to administer these tests to their clients. Additionally, counselors with bilingual clients should check with their clients to determine which language their clients are most proficient in and administer tests in that language.

Environmental Influences on Career Testing

In addition to cultural factors, environmental factors such as the pitfalls of socioeconomic status, the effects of community support, or lack thereof, on individuals, and the effects of racism and discrimination on individuals may influence career testing results.

Socioeconomic Status

As stated previously, differences in test scores within cultural groups can be directly related to socioeconomic status. Poverty is likely to result in poor physical health, poor nutrition, and poor cognitive development—all of which affect the results of aptitude tests (Neisser et al., 1996). Moreover, poverty correlates with inadequate educational preparation, further affecting the test scores of clients from poor socioeconomic backgrounds (Krane & Tirre, 2005). Inadequate education and preparation subsequently lead to lower-level occupation options, unemployment, and, for some, criminal activity. As far as testing is concerned, counselors should be aware of the academic limitations of their clients before administering tests. For example, the counselor should be aware of the client's reading level and obtain an appropriate form of the test, if one is available, or make other adaptations, such as employing a reader.

School districts with limited resources, such as those in impoverished areas, may not have room in the budget for a battery of tests. Counselors would do well to discover testing resources at reasonable costs to the district—perhaps hand-scored tests rather than computer-scored ones, tests that allow for the duplication of a certain number of forms, and lower-cost online assessments that counselors may want to take advantage of. Whatever the clientele, counselors need to be creative and resourceful when they choose to use standardized testing, but the demands of frugality are particularly strong in economically struggling school districts.

Community

The community is another environmental factor that may influence test outcomes. In cultures that are more collaborative than others, community support may be extensive. In a collaborative community, an individual's interest inventory or aptitude test may be either supported by the community or not. A well-used analogy compares people in a community to crabs in a barrel. The crabs on the bottom are always pulling the crabs crawling to the top back down to the bottom. This analogy carries through to Gottfredson's (1981) theory of circumscription, in which the author suggests that individuals often give up on career options that would require too much effort to achieve or would be unacceptable in their communities. On the other hand, supportive communities, acting in unison to uplift young people, may encourage careers that students may have felt out of their reach. Some high school students, for example, have attended SAT preparation courses at their churches and community centers. Career-development programs sponsored by clergy, politicians, businesses, and so forth that are inclusive of community members have been known to have a positive effect on the career options of young people, and these young people may express wider career interests on their inventory interest results (D'Andrea & Daniels, 1992).

Racism and Discrimination

Racism and discrimination may also influence client attitudes toward career testing. Subich (1996) has suggested using Swanson and Tokar's (1991) Career Barriers Inventory to help determine the degree to which clients believe they are limited in their careers as a result of racism and discrimination. Administering the Career Barriers Inventory to multicultural populations facilitates discussion between the client and counselor and provides counselors with greater insight into the effects of racism and discrimination on their clients. Unfortunately, client perceptions of barriers may affect client willingness to participate in career testing. Some clients may have had such extensive negative experiences with testing while attending school that they "may not trust and therefore may be suspicious of the assessment process" (Gainor, 2000, p. 180).

Racism and discrimination in employment testing is still a problem, albeit to a lesser degree than in the past, according to Drummond and Jones (2006). At one time, career tests were used to eliminate individuals from jobs due to their demographic attributes, such as race, gender, age, and so forth. Nowadays, one would hope that such practices are unheard of. However, until racism and discrimination no longer exist in our society, such practices may persist, perhaps in less overtly intentional ways, but persist nonetheless via culturally encapsulated test creators, administrators, and career counselors.

Cultural and Environmental Factors Applied to Malachi's Situation

The following continuation of the Malachi vignette reveals Malachi's cultural and environmental situation. In order for his counselor, Jim, to effectively administer and interpret Malachi's test results, he will need to take these cultural and environmental factors into consideration:

In terms of culture, Malachi's family has taught him to be proud of his cultural heritage. He attends a black church regularly and participates in the church's youth group, but this is not his primary recreation. Included in his cultural education about African Americans is a sense of responsibility to give back to his community and to value good works. Malachi and his immediate family always speak Standard English unless emphasis is needed on a particular point, in which case they may employ Black Vernacular English. Many family members outside of their household tend to switch between Standard English and Black Vernacular depending on who is being addressed. Malachi lives in an extended family household. He is the oldest of three children—he has two sisters. His father died when Malachi was nine years old, at which time his maternal grandmother (also a widow) came to live with them. About a year ago, Malachi's mother's second cousin, Aisha (two years his junior), came to live with them as well, because Aisha's mother was deployed to the war in Iraq. Malachi says that living with five women hasn't been difficult, except when they hog the bathroom or badmouth black men.

In terms of racial identity, Malachi is in the dissonance stage, moving toward the resistance stage. Malachi is just waking up to the reality of racism against African American males. He had read about it, and he had been taught about the history of discrimination, but until he and his friends grew to their current height, racism was an abstract concept to Malachi. Now when he walks down the street with four or five of his friends, they are eyed warily and scrutinized by other people. Malachi's uncle had told him once about the problems of being stopped by law enforcement officers for DWB (Driving While Black), and Malachi had laughed. Now he doesn't think the DWB concept is so funny anymore.

In terms of environment, Malachi lives in a working-class neighborhood that is predominantly African American. Several children in the neighborhood have gone to college (most to the local community college), and Malachi is feeling the pressure to go as well. In fact, his mother is always hassling him about it. From Malachi's career genogram (career family tree), Malachi's career counselor Jim discovers that the men in Malachi's family have traditionally been skilled workers—mechanics, brick masons, carpenters, and so forth. The women have been nurses and domestic workers. Malachi's father and paternal grandfather were mechanics, but Malachi is not interested in that work, because his father died in a freak accident at work. Malachi's mother is an administrative assistant at a book publishing company.

Jim uses the information about Malachi's cultural background not only to determine the appropriate tests for the client but also to interpret those tests. If he goes to college, Malachi will be the first one in his family to do so. It is important that Jim repeatedly caution Malachi that the tests are not infallible but in fact, because of the low percentages of individuals to compare him against, they may not give a truly accurate snapshot of Malachi. Jim will want to assess Malachi's racial identity status because it may have a great impact on his career interests and the career decisions he makes later. Malachi appears to be between identity stages, and it would be helpful if Jim could see Malachi's profile. Jim will need to recall when he interprets the results of the interest and ability testing how important family and community are to Malachi. Giving back to the community is a very significant value that will be reflected in several of Malachi's tests. Finally Jim should keep in mind that Malachi's male family history is overwhelmingly blue collar—a fact that may show up in Malachi's interests inventory and test results. Jim will need to address this phenomenon with Malachi during interpretation as well.

TEST INTERPRETATION FOR DIVERSE POPULATIONS

Prior to interpretation of test results, counselors should already have been culturally sensitive and diligent in the selection of appropriate tests for their clients, and may already have performed qualitative assessments to establish rapport, defined the career problems, gathered information about the client's culture and level of acculturation, and determined that formal testing is the best option to unearth the information the client needs. Qualitative assessment may include interview questions, career stories, career fantasies, guided imagery, and so forth. Many authors recommend that qualitative assessment be given to all culturally different populations (Highlen & Sudarsky-Gleiser, 1994; Goldman, 1990). They argue that there are too many possible pitfalls with the use of standardized testing, and therefore qualitative assessment is a necessary step in avoiding stereotyping and labeling clients. To get a true measure of the client's possible career testing pitfalls and to insure that tests are not interpreted in a culturally encapsulated manner, multiple qualitative assessments should be administered. Comas-Diaz (1996) lists twenty factors that counselors should consider discussing with culturally different clients in a pretesting interview. In addition to the topics discussed in previous chapters such as race, racial identity, culture, religion, socioeconomic status and history, sexual orientation and physical disabilities, and interests, she also suggests discussing historical age cohorts, acculturation, experiences with trauma and abuse, marital status, and genetic dispositions. Not every factor will need to be discussed with every client.

Taking all Comas-Diaz's factors into consideration is a daunting task, however. An additional daunting factor for counselors, as Ridley, Li, and Hill (1998) point out, is that the career counseling literature consistently recommends that counselors consider factors of culture and environment, yet rarely does the literature give guidance about how to do so. It is not surprising that beginning career counselors may feel overwhelmed with the responsibility. In an effort to help, several authors have designed models for multicultural career assessment, two of which are discussed in more detail below: the Ridley, Li, and Hill model, and the model of Flores and colleagues.

Models of Multicultural and Career Assessment

The Ridley, Li, and Hill model and the model of Flores and colleagues have been designed to assist the multicultural career counselor to synthesize cultural information and make decisions about how to use cultural information. Neither model is explicit regarding selecting, administering, and interpreting tests. However both of the models provide some structure for utilizing both qualitative and quantitative data gleaned from the client.

The Ridley, Li, and Hill Model: The Multicultural Assessment Process (MAP)

Ridley, Li, and Hill offer a conceptual framework, known as the Multicultural Assessment Process, or MAP, for assessment that they say is missing from previous multicultural testing literature. While these authors developed their MAP model to focus on the assessment of psychological disorders, the model is readily adaptable for career counselors. Figure 6.2 lists MAP's ten foundational principles. These principles include not only the need to thoroughly assess culture and environment, but also to take this need one step further into practical application by speaking to the complexity and subjectivity of the cultural/environmental assessment process.

According to Ridley, Li, and Hill, most of all clinical assessment needs "a systematic methodology based on a conceptually coherent framework" (p. 858). As a result, the Multicultural Assessment Process (MAP) is systematically organized into a four-phase framework: (1) identify cultural data, (2) interpret cultural data, (3) incorporate cultural data, and (4) arrive at a sound assessment decision. Ridley, Li, and Hill also provide "decision points" throughout the process—decisions that need to be made to keep the process on track. In addition, the authors include debiasing strategies to assist counselors in making good decisions.

Figure 6.2   Foundational Principles of MAP

1. A sound assessment is accurate and comprehensive (p. 853).
2. Assessment is a larger concept than is diagnostic classification [and] . . . includes prognosis, severity ratings, compilation of strengths and resources, and social supports (pp. 853–854).
3. Psychological assessment is complex (p. 854).
4. Psychological assessment is a process of progressive decision making (p. 854).
5. As a decision-making process, assessment involves considerable subjectivity (p. 855).
6. A sound assessment has clinical utility (p. 857).
7. Culture is always relevant to psychological assessment (p. 857).
8. Assessment should include dispositional and environmental factors (p. 858).
9. Sound assessment requires a systematic methodology based on a conceptually coherent framework (p. 858).
10. Psychological assessment is a challenging responsibility (pp. 853–859).[1]

[1] Table cites section headings for the pages listed.

Phase 1 of MAP is to identify the client's cultural information, whether this information seems relevant or not, and Phase 2 involves interpreting and organizing to yield a "working hypothesis" (p. 873) about the possible origins of a client's problems with choosing a career, with the goal of testing this hypothesis as valid or invalid during Phase 3. In other words, Ridley, Li, and Hill suggest that counselors develop a scientific attitude. They suggest that counselors "use psychological testing to test hypotheses, not to generate them" (p. 881).

This is an interesting idea in career counseling. For example, if a counselor hypothesizes that client A's career interests differ greatly from those her parents wish her to pursue, the counselor would administer an interest test to prove or disprove that hypothesis. As a result, the interpretation of the test results may be more relevant to the test taker. This procedure also forces counselors to think about and choose tests more methodically. During this phase, the counselor should also be aware of biases in testing and should be alert to test interpretation, especially concerning statistical error and the standard error of measurement.

Finally, in Phase 4 of MAP, the counselor uses information gleaned from hypothesis testing to make a final decision or diagnosis to help the client move forward. For example, if the results of Client A's interest inventory prove the hypothesis, suggesting that the client does, in fact, have different interests from those her parents wish her to pursue, then the next step would be discuss these differences with the client and perhaps bring in her parents, if it is appropriate for her cultural group, to discuss these differences. For some clients, differences between their career ideas and their parents' may not be such an issue. Then, it would be appropriate to introduce the client to other similar-minded people, who may act as her role models. Sometimes the counselor may need to recycle through the MAP process, based on the results of hypothesis testing—for example if the hypothesis does not stand up to testing. However, Ridley and colleagues (1998) warn counselors not to get caught up in endless testing and retesting cycles. In addition, Ridley et al. (1998) recommend using "debiasing" techniques during the MAP process to ensure that assessments have not been compromised by counselor values and beliefs regarding their clients' cultures. Counselors may erroneously employ one of three possible heuristics that impede scientific judgment: (a) failing to search for further information because the answer seems obvious based on the counselor's experience with similar client problems (known as the "availability heuristic"); (b) favoring information given at the beginning of an interview and ignoring information given later on (known as the "anchoring heuristic"); and (c) relying on stereotypes when looking for norms among a client's cultural group (known as the "representativeness heuristic"). To combat these errors, Ridley and colleagues recommend the following debiasing strategies to combat these heuristics:

- Looking for other explanations for client problems, such as environmental or cultural explanations, rather than relying on stereotypes or past experiences with other clients (Arkes, 1981).
- Reframing interpretations of client issues so that they speak to strengths rather than weaknesses (for example, the client with few resources due to

low socioeconomic status, but who is still successful may be referred to as resourceful rather than disadvantaged).

- Delaying making a decision about client issues in order to increase objectivity. This is a process similar to holding onto an emotion-packed letter for three days to cool off before mailing (Spengler et al., 1995).

The Flores, Spanierman, and Obasi Model: Culturally Appropriate Career Assessment Model (CACAM)

In their discussion of test selection, Flores, Spanierman, and Obasi (2003) provide recommendations to test developers and researchers that will assist counselors to administer tests with diverse populations. Among other things, Flores, Spanierman, and Obasi suggest that when test developers see performance differences among diverse groups, developers need to scientifically construct scales to accurately measure diverse groups. In addition, Flores and colleagues stress that counselors and psychologists need to establish their own reliability and validity data for specific populations, and that more representative samples need to be used in normative data. The authors suggest the use of qualitative assessment, nonstandard tests, computers, and verbal methods; they also advocate taking career assessment out into the community: to churches, community centers, and schools.

The CACAM assumes that counselors are competent in general, career, and multicultural counseling. There are four steps in the CACAM. (1) "information gathering, (2) selection of career instruments, (3) administration of career instruments (4) interpretation of career assessments results" (p. 81). Flores, Spanierman, and Obasi believe that much can be discovered from sources other than standardized testing such as interviewing the client and following up with information taken from intake forms, checklists, and inventories that measure worldview and cultural values.

Not only do Flores, Spanierman, and Obasi discuss the issues of widely used standardized tests such as the Strong Interest Inventory, they also recommend that counselors review career tests for problems with test construction regarding cultural validity and equivalency (linguistic, conceptual, scale, and normative equivalence). Only after such a review should a counselor administer a test. Of course, the next step would be the culturally appropriate administration of the selected tests that requires a strong relationship with the client and an environment that is welcoming and safe to the client, and everything should be done to make the environment comfortable including adjusting the physical accommodations or hiring readers.

The last step is the culturally appropriate interpretation of tests. Flores, Spanierman, and Obasi (2003) are similar to Ridley and colleagues in that they suggest using client information to test hypotheses about client testing needs and assessments. According to Flores and colleagues, counselors need to look for consistencies in the data—both qualitative and quantitative—before making hypotheses. In their view, integrating cultural data with testing data is essential, and any information communicated to clients should be in a format clients will readily understand.

Test Interpretation as Applied to Malachi's Situation

The following is a summary of sections of Jim's interpretation of Malachi's scores—the sections that address the integration of culture and environment into the interpretation. Jim has administered the SAT, the Strong Interest Inventory, and the 16PF personality test to Malachi.

SAT

Malachi, before you took the SAT, we talked about what you wanted to get from taking this test, and as I recall, you wanted to get an idea of whether or not you were "college material." Is that still what you wanted to know? (They discuss the goals for taking this test and Malachi's reaction to the test itself.) We also talked about some of the issues for African Americans regarding the results. You may recall that African Americans have traditionally scored lower than whites on the SAT. There have been a great many debates as to why this occurs, but no definitive proven reasons have been found. What we do know is that the SAT is good at predicting college performance for African Americans as well as whites. Your score of 1250 (690 verbal, 560 quantitative) indicates that you have great potential to be successful in college. I was worried that your scores may have been negatively affected after our talk about how African Americans score lower than whites. At least that is my understanding of what sometimes happens. But you did very well. In fact, you scored in a range that indicates that you could probably have done better in high school than you have. What is your reaction to that? (Jim goes on to explore this issue with Malachi.) So it seems you could be making As and Bs, but maybe you think this would make you uncool. (Malachi agrees that he doesn't want to seem too smart, or his friends will give him grief about it. Jim empathizes and asks how his friends will feel about his going to college. Malachi replies that they will probably be cool with it. They have other friends who have gone to college and Malachi thinks his friends respect them for it.) So, college is cool but being a geek is not. Jim then suggested that his family and his church would be very happy if he went to college and did well. Malachi agreed and said that it was what his mother had been pushing for the last year, but he really didn't think he had a chance to get in. Jim said, "Malachi, with your GPA you will probably be more competitive right now at the community-college level, but we should leave the four-year college option open, because your SAT scores are good, and depending on what you intend to take as your major and how you feel about being at a more hectic and competitive four-year institution, you could perform well at a four-year college as well. Remember what I said about how SAT scores tend to over-predict performance for African American men? What that means is that you may not get as high of a Grade Point Average as your white classmates with the same SAT scores. Tell me, what is your reaction to this information?" (Malachi says that if he gets into college, he won't fool around as he did in his high school classes, so he will probably have a good GPA.)

During this interpretation, Jim did a good job of including Malachi in the conversation about the results. He reminded Malachi of the limitations of the test for African Americans but, most importantly, Jim took into consideration the reactions of Malachi's family and friends.

Strong Interest Inventory

(They first discuss the reason for taking the Strong Interest Inventory.) "Malachi, you may remember that we decided on the Strong Interest Inventory to give you some ideas about careers you may not be aware of that may interest you. I feel pretty confident about some of your results on the Strong Interest Inventory. Remember that we discussed that the Strong Interest Inventory was researched very heavily to see how it works with African Americans. The general occupational themes tend not to vary in terms of people's ethnicity, so when I give you your results on the General Occupational Themes, you can feel pretty certain that they are not biased against African Americans. (Jim goes on to report on the GOTs.)*

The Basic Interest Scales and the Occupational scales have not been proven scientifically to differentiate among cultural groups, so we really don't know, for example, whether you are similar to other African Americans in nuclear engineering or any other career field. What will show is how similar you are to a general population of nuclear engineers (whether they are white, black, Asian, or any other group). You may have similar interests as these individuals, and you may not. We just don't have that kind of comparison information right now. We decided to go on with this test because we thought it would give us a better idea of the general categories of careers that you might be interested in. I think it has done that. (Jim goes on to report Malachi's results on the Basic Interest and Occupational scales, paying particular attention to the careers Malachi has shown an interest in and that reflect some of his family interests, such as mechanical engineering. Malachi may look at other engineering types of jobs as well as those related to the field that do not require four years of college.)

Again, Jim is meticulous about reminding Malachi about why the test was chosen and the limitations of the test for African Americans. What is not included here is Jim's discussion of traditional careers for African Americans. Jim was concerned that Malachi may score similar to and want to limit his career choices to those traditional careers. Such a discussion is appropriate when interpreting the result of an interest inventory—based on stereotypic careers groupings.

16 PF

Remember that this is a personality test, and it will give us some information about your personality characteristics that might be helpful in selecting a career. Some of the things in your culture that you say are important are your family, your connection with other African Americans, and the fact that you want to make both your family and the people in your community proud of you. Some of these values are reflected in this inventory. Now, the 16PF did a much better job at getting ethnic minority participation than the SII. The group you are compared against (the normative sample) are represented in proportion to their numbers in the general U.S. population. The U.S. population is 12 percent African American, and 12 percent of the people your scores are compared against are African Americans. Interestingly, they didn't find any real differences between African Americans and other groups on most of the scales of the 16PF. However, in this new version, there is a general reasoning scale (which is an ability measure), and African Americans score lower on that scale than whites. We really do not need the reasoning scale because you have already taken the SAT and that is a good measure of your abilities. (Jim goes on to report Malachi's 16PF scores.) One more thing, remember that your score is supposed to reflect what you were like on a typical day. People change, and their test scores on personality tests are likely to be affected by those changes, but usually in personality tests, the scores are pretty stable. Even so, these tests are not 100 percent precise as compared to, say a DNA test. If you were to take the test again, for example, you might get the same score, but it is more likely that your scores will fall within a certain range, and we can be pretty confident about that range by using a statistical formula.

Jim did a good job again reminding Malachi about the purpose and limitations of the test. He was careful to mention how Malachi's family and community helped contribute to his personality development and how that would be reflected in the test results.

FINAL THOUGHTS ABOUT TESTING

Testing/assessment is a technical and complicated process that causes anxiety for both clients and counselors. Although it is always inadvisable to offer cookbook solutions to complicated issues, it may help to summarize some of the research described in this chapter. With that in mind, following are some guidelines for administering tests to culturally diverse groups in career counseling:

1. Review the purpose of tests collaboratively with clients to ensure that the tests utilized will meet client needs.
2. If the test seems to meet client needs, investigate the test by reading all available information about its cultural inclusiveness (such as manuals, mental measurements yearbooks, research articles), including information on language and reading levels.
3. Pay special attention to the standardization sample. Ensure that diversity percentages are close to population numbers of diverse groups. If there are *no* ethnic minorities listed among the normative sample, justify the use of this particular test with a particular client (justifications might include that the client is highly acculturated or that local norms exist for the test).
4. If the test *utilizes* ethnic minorities or other special populations in the normative sample, pay close attention to how close the ethnic population compares to that of the U.S. general population. Also, check to see if any analyses have been conducted comparing the responses of different cultural groups. If the ethnic population numbers are too small and/or there is no cultural comparison data, administration of the test needs to be justified, as in item 3 above.
5. If there is data concerning testing differences between culturally different groups, note the data and make a decision as to whether or not to proceed with testing. If there are norms for your client's group, it is feasible to go ahead and use the test. If there are testing differences, but no norms for your client's cultural group, the information about the norming sample may still be used to interpret a client's test results. Determine how this information will be reported to the client.

6. Always explain to clients any caveats before administering you interpret the test for clients.

7. Provide the best interpretation of the test results you ca ation the client's race, culture, and environment. Son helpful are:

(a) We decided to use this test because . . .

(b) This test has limitations for you because . . . What do you think?

(c) A few of the things that are important to you as a _____ are . . . and this test _____. Am I right?

(d) What all this means for you, according to what you have told me, is _____. Does that sound right to you?

REVIEW/REFLECTION QUESTIONS

1. Use either the Flores, Spanierman, and Obasi Model or the Ridley, Hill, & Li Model, to assess your own career development. Discuss each of the steps and how each one may be useful in helping a client like yourself who is experiencing career problems.

2. Given the criticisms of cultural relevance of testing, how do you see psychological testing changing in the next twenty years as the United States becomes a more diverse country?

3. Review the guidelines in the last section of the chapter. Create a list of Don'ts (things not to do) for administering and interpreting tests with culturally different groups.

4. You have been asked to create a culturally fair math aptitude test based on the information in this chapter. What are some of the cultural issues you should be aware of when creating this test? How will you solve these cultural dilemmas in your test?

REFERENCES

American Counseling Association (ACA) (2005). ACA Code of Ethics. Retrieved *http://www.counseling.org/Resources/CodeOfEthics/TP/Home/CT2.aspx*

Anderson, M. Z.,Tracey, T. J. G. & Rounds, J. (1997). Examining the invariance of Holland's vocational interest model across gender. *Journal of vocational behavior, 50,* 349–364.

Association for Assessment in Counseling and Education (2003). Standards for Multicultural Assessment. Retrieved December 4, 2006 from *http://aac.ncat.edu/Resources/documents/STANDARDS%20FOR%20MULTICULTURAL%20ASSESSMENT%20FINAL.pdf*

@Arkes, H. R. (1981). Impediments to accurate clinical judgment and possible ways tominimize their impact. *Journal of Consulting and Clinical Psychology, 49,* 323–330. Association for Assessment in Counseling, Author (2003). (*http://aac.ncat.edu/resources/documents/STANDARDS%20FOR%20MULTICULTURAL%20ASSESSMENT%20FINAL.pdf*) retrieved 8/14/06.

Arredondo, P., Toporek, R., Brown, S. P., Jones, J., Locke, D. C., Sanchez, J., & Stadler, H. (1996). Operationalization of the multicultural counseling competencies. *Journal of Multicultural Counseling and Development, 24*, 42–78.

Atkinson, D. R., & Gim, R.H. (1989). Asian American cultural identity and attitudes toward mental health services. *The Journal of Counseling Psychology, 36*(2), 209–212.

Berry, J. W. (1980). Acculturation as varieties of adaptation. In A. Padilla (Ed.), Westview Press.

Betz, N. E. (1992). Counseling uses of self-efficacy theory. *Career Development Quarterly, 41*, 22–26.

Betz, N. E., & Hackett, G. (1987). The concept of agency in educational and career development. *Journal of Counseling Psychology, 34*, 311–320.

Carter, R. T., & Swanson, J. L. (1990). The validity of the Strong Interest Inventory with Black Americans: A review of the literature. *Journal of Vocational Behavior, 36*, 195–209.

Chartrand, J. M., & Walsh, W. B. (2001). Career assessment: Changes and trends. In F. T. L. Leong & A. Barak (Eds.), *Contemporary models in vocational psychology* (pp. 231–255). Mahwah, NJ: Lawrence Erlbaum.

Chung, Y. B., & Harmon, L. W. (1994). The career interests and aspirations of gay men: How sex-role orientation is related. *Journal of Vocational Behavior, 45*(2), 223–239.

College Board (n.d.). CollegeBoard connect to college success. Retrieved March 2, 2006 from the World Wide Web, http://www.collegeboard.com/splash.

Comas-Diaz, L. (1996). Cultural considerations in diagnosis. In F. W. Kaslow (Ed.), *Handbook on Relational Diagnosis and Dysfunctional Family Patterns* (pp. 152–168). Oxford, England: John Wiley, & Sons, Inc.

Constantine, M. G. (1998). Developing competence in multicultural assessment: Implications for counseling psychology training and practice. *Counseling Psychologist, 26*(6), 922–929.

Croteau, J. M., Anderson, M. Z., & Distefano, T. M. (2000). Lesbian, gay, and bisexual vocational psychology: Reviewing foundations and planning construction. In: R. M. Perez, K. A. DeBord, & K. J. Bieschke (Eds*). Handbook of counseling and psychotherapy with lesbian, gay, and bisexual clients* (pp. 383–408). Washington, DC, US: American Psychological Association.

D'Andrea, M., & Daniels, J. (1992). A career development program for inner-city Black youth. *Career Development Quarterly, 40*(3), 272–280.

Day, S. X., & Rounds, J. (1998). Universality of vocational interest structure among racial and ethnic minorities. *American Psychologist, 53*(7), 728–736.

DeWitt, D. W. (1994). Using the Strong with people who have disabilities. In L. W.Harmon, Hansen, J., & Borgen, F. H. *Strong Interest Inventory: Applications and Technical Guide* (pp. 281–290). Stanford, CA: Stanford University Press.

Drummond, R. J. & Jones, K. D. (2006). *Assessment procedures for counselors and helping professions* (6th Ed.). Upper Saddle River, NJ: Pearson Education Inc.

Fleming, J. (2000). Affirmative action and standardized test scores. *Journal of Negro Education, 69*(1–2), 27–37.

Flores, L. Y., Spanierman, L. B., & Obasi, E. M. (2003). Ethical and professional issues in career assessment with diverse racial and ethnic groups. *Journal of Career Assessment, 11*, 76–95.

Fouad, N A., Harmon, L. W., & Borgen, F. H. (1997). Structure of interests in employed male and female members of US racial-ethnic minority and nonminority groups. *Journal of Counseling Psychology, 44*, 339–345.

Freedle, R. O. (2003) Correcting the SAT's ethnic and social-class bias: A method for reestimating SAT scores. *Harvard Educational Review, 73*, 1–43.

Freeman, K. (1997). Increasing African American's participation in higher education: African American high school students' perpectives. *Journal of Higher Education, 68,* 523–550.

Freeman, K. (1999). The race factor in African American's college choice. *Urban Education, 34,* 4–25.

Fukuyama, M. A., & Cox, C. I. (1992). Asian-Pacific Islanders and career development. In D. Brown & C. Minor (Eds.), *Career needs in a diverse workforce: Implications of the NCDA Gallup survey* (pp. 27–50). Alexandria, VA: National Career Development Association.

Hackett, G., & Lonborg, S. D. (1993). Career assessment and counseling for women. In W. B. Walsh & S. H. Osipow (Eds.), *Career counseling for women* (pp. 43–85). Hillsdale, N.J.: Erlbaum.

Hansen, J. I. C. (1987) Cross-cultural research on vocational interests. *Measurement and Evaluation in Counseling and Development, 20,* 65–71.

Harmon, L. W., Hansen, J. C., Borgen, F., & Hammer, A. (1994). *Strong Interest Inventory: Application and Technical Guide.* Palo Alto, CA: Consulting Psychologists Press.

Hartman, N. S., McDaniel, M. A, & Whetzel, D. L. (2003). Gender, race, and ethnic differences on assessment tools used in career guidance and counseling. In J. Wall & G. Walz (Eds.), *Measuring Up: The Ultimate Resource on Testing for Teachers, Counselors, and Administrators.* Greensboro, NC: ERIC/CASS and NBCC. 99–105.

Healy, C. C. (1990). Reforming career appraisals to meet the needs of clients in the 1990s. *Counseling Psychologist, 18,* 214–226.

Helms, J. E. (1992). Why is there no study of cultural equivalence in standardized cognitive ability testing? *American Psychologist, 47*(9), 1083–1101.

Herrnstein, R. J., & Murray, C. (1994). *The Bell Curve.* New York: The Free Press.

Highlen, P. S., & Sudarsky-Gleiser, C. (1994). Co-Essence Model of Vocational Assessment for Racial/Ethnic Minorities (CEMVA-REM): An existential model. *Journal of Career Assessment, 2,* 304–329.

Hofstede, G. (1986). Cultural differences in teaching and learning. *International Journal of Intercultural Relations, 10,* 301–320.

Gainor, K. A. (2000). Vocational assessment with culturally diverse populations. In L. A. Suzuki, J. G. Ponterotto & P. J. Meller (Eds.), *Handbook of multicultural assessment: Clinical, psychological, and educational applications* (2nd ed.) (pp. 169–189). San Francisco, CA: Jossey-Bass.

Gainor, K. A., & Lent, R. W. (1998). Social cognitive expectations and racial identity attitudes in predicting the math choice intentions of Black college students. *Journal of Counseling Psychology, 45,* 403–413

Goldman, L. (1990). Qualitative assessment. *The Counseling Psychologist, 18*(2), 205–213.

Gottfredson, L. S. (1981). Circumscription and compromise: A developmental theory of occupational aspirations. *Journal of Counseling Psychology (Monograph), 28* (6), 545–579.

Gottfredson, G. D., & Holland, J. L. (1975). Vocational choices of men and women: A comparison of predictors from the Self-Directed Search. *Journal of Counseling Psychology, 22*(1), 28–34.

Holland, J. L. (1997). *Making vocational choices: A theory of vocational personality and work environments* (3rd ed.). Odessa, FL: Psychological Assessment Resources.

Jensen, A. R. (1980). *Bias in mental testing.* New York, NY: Free Press.

Jensen, A. R. (1998). *The g factor: The science of mental ability.* Westport, CT: Praeger/Greenwood.

Kapes, J. T., & Martinez, L. (1999). Career assessment with special populations: A survey of national experts. Paper presented at the annual meeting of the Association for Career and Technology Education, Orlando, Florida.

Kelly, K. R. (2003). Review of the Strong Interest Inventory. In B. S. Plake, J. C. Impara, & R. A. Spies (Eds.), *The fifteenth mental measurements yearbook* (pp. 894–897). Lincoln, NE: Buros Institute of Mental Measurements.

Krane, N. E. R., & Tirre, W. C. (2005). Ability Assessment in Career Counseling. In S. D. Brown & R. W. Lent (Eds.). *Career development and counseling: Putting theory and research to work* (pp. 330–352). Hoboken, NJ: John Wiley & Sons, Inc.

LaFramboise, T. D., Trimble, J. E., & Mohatt, G. V. (1990). Counseling intervention and American Indian tradition. *The Counseling Psychologist, 18*, 628–654.

Lee, C. C. (1997). Cultural dynamics: Their importance in culturally responsive counseling. In C. C. Lee (Ed.), *Multicultural issues in counseling: New approaches to diversity* (2nd ed., pp. 15–30). Alexandria, VA: American Counseling Association.

Lee, C. C., & Chuang, B. (2005). Counseling people of color. In D. Capuzzi & D. R. Gross (Eds.), *Introduction to the Counseling Profession.* (pp. 465–483). New York: Allyn & Bacon.

Levine, E. S., & Padilla, A. M. (1980). *Crossing Cultures in Therapy: Pluralistic Counseling for the Hispanic.* Monterey, CA: Brooks/Cole.

Loehlin, J. C., Lindzey, G., & Spuhler, J. N. (1975). *Race differences in intelligence.* San Francisco: Freeman.

Meir, E. I., & Tziner, A. (2001). Cross-cultural assessment of interests. In F. T. L. Leong & A. Barak (Eds.), *Contemporary models in vocational psychology* (pp. 133–166). Mahwah, NJ: Erlbaum.

Mobley, M., & Slaney, R. B. (1996). Holland's theory: Its relevance for lesbian and gay career clients. *Journal of Vocational Behavior, 48*, 125–135.

NCDA (author) (1997). Career Counseling Competencies. Retrieved August 16, 2006, from *http://www.ncda.org/pdf/counselingcompetencies.pdf*

Neisser, U., Boodoo, G., Bouchard, T. J., Boykin, A. W., Brody, N., Ceci, S. J., Halpern, D. F., Loehlin, J. C., Perloff, R., Sternberg, R. J., & Urbina, S. (1996). Intelligence: Knowns and unknowns. *American Psychologist, 51*(2), 77–101.

Niles, S. G., & Harris-Bowlsbey, J. (2005). *Introduction to career development interventions in the 21st century* (2nd edition) Columbus, OH: Merrill Prentice Hall.

Olmedo, E. L., & Padilla, A. M. (1978). Empirical and construct validation of a measure of acculturation for Mexican Americans, *Journal of Social Psychology, 10,* 179–187.

Ridley, C. R., Li, L. C., & Hill, C. L. (1998). Multicultural assessment: Reexamination, reconceptualization, and practical application. *The Counseling Psychologist, 26*(6), 939–947.

Ryan-Krane, N. E., & Tirre, W. C. (2005). Ability assessment in career counseling. In S. D. Brown & R.W. Lent (Eds.), *Career development and counseling: Putting theory and research to work* (pp. 330–352). Hoboken, NJ: John Wiley & Sons, Inc.

Spengler, P. M., Strohmer, D. C., & Dixon, D. N. (1995). A scientist-practitioner model of psychological assessment: Implications for training, practice and research. *Counseling Psychologist, 23*, 506–534.

Steele, C. M., & Aronson, J. (1995). Stereotype threat and the intellectual test performance of African Americans. *Journal of Personality and Social Psychology, 69*, 797–811.

Subich, L. M. (1996). Addressing diversity in the process of career assessment. In M. L. Savickas & W. B. Walsh (Eds.), *Handbook of career counseling theory and practice* (pp. 277–289). Palo Alto, CA: Davies-Black.

Swanson, J. L., & Tokar, D. M. (1991). Development and initial validation of the Career Barriers Inventory. *Journal of Vocational Behavior, 39,* 344–361.

Thomason, T. C. (1999). Psychological and vocational assessment of Native Americans. ERIC document *http://www.eric.ed.gov/ERICDocs/data/ericdocs2/content_storage_01/0000000b/80/11/9a/c4.pdf.* Retrieved August 16, 2006.

Walpole, M., McDonough, P. M., & Bauer, C. J. (2005). This Test is Unfair: Urban African American and Latino High School Students' Perceptions of Standardized College Admission Tests. *Urban Education, 40,* 321–349.

Whitcomb, D. H., Wettersten, K. B., & Stolz, C. L. (2006). Career counseling with gay, lesbian, bisexual and transgender clients. In D. Capuzzi & M. S. Stauffer (Eds.). *Career Counseling: Foundations, Perspectives, and Applications* (386–420). Boston: Allyn and Bacon.

CHAPTER 7
Multiculturally Competent Career Counseling Skills

Career development texts typically cover a broad spectrum of topics that help readers to understand what career development is without focusing on counseling skills, which are central to the success of the process of career development. Career counselors can learn how to access and communicate to clients the seemingly endless amount of information available about careers and about the career decision-making process, but if career counselors do not possess the skills to work effectively with people, including people from diverse backgrounds, their clients will not be able to effectively process all of the information they have been given. Therefore, to further help counselors acquire both the career counseling and multicultural counseling skills they need to work effectively with all populations, this chapter will integrate the National Career Development Association Guidelines for Individual and Group Counseling Skills (NCDA, 1997) with the relevant Association for Multicultural Counseling and Development (AMCD) competencies (Arredondo et al., 1996; Roysircar et al., 2003), both of which were outlined in Chapter 1 of this book and are reiterated in Figures 7.1 and 7.2 below. Then, the integrated competencies will be applied to the seven stages of the counseling process, with a case example woven into the discussion to illustrate the process more concretely.

Figure 7.1   NCDA Career Counseling Competencies—Individual and Group Counseling Skills

1. Establish and maintain productive personal relationships with individuals
2. Establish and maintain a productive group environment
3. Collaborate with clients in identifying personal goals
4. Identify and select techniques appropriate to client or group goals and client needs, psychological states, and developmental tasks
5. Identify and understand clients' personal characteristics related to career
6. Identify and understand social contextual conditions affecting clients' careers
7. Identify and understand familial, subcultural, and cultural structures as they are related to clients' careers
8. Identify and understand clients' career decision-making processes
9. Identify and understand clients' attitudes toward work and workers
10. Identify and understand clients' biases toward work and workers based on gender, race, and cultural stereotypes
11. Challenge and encourage clients to take action to prepare for and initiate role transitions by locating sources of relevant information and experience, obtaining and interpreting information and experiences, and acquiring skills needed to make role transitions
12. Assist the client to acquire a set of employability and job search skills
13. Support and challenge clients to examine life-work roles, including the balance of work, leisure, family and community in their careers (NCDA, 1997).

Reproduced with permission from NCDA.

Figure 7.2   AMCD Multicultural Counseling Competencies

I. Counselor Awareness of Own Cultural Values and Biases
  A. Attitudes and Beliefs
    1. Culturally skilled counselors believe that cultural self-awareness and sensitivity to one's own cultural heritage is essential.
    2. Culturally skilled counselors are aware of how their own cultural background and experiences have influenced attitudes, values, and biases about psychological processes.
    3. Culturally skilled counselors are able to recognize the limits of their multicultural competency and expertise.
    4. Culturally skilled counselors recognize their sources of discomfort with differences that exist between themselves and clients in terms of race, ethnicity, and culture.

  B. Knowledge
    1. Culturally skilled counselors have specific knowledge about their own racial and cultural heritage and how it personally and professionally affects their definitions of and biases about normality/abnormality and the process of counseling.
    2. Culturally skilled counselors possess knowledge and understanding about how oppression, racism, discrimination, and stereotyping affect them personally and in their work. This allows individuals to acknowledge their own racist attitudes, beliefs, and feelings. Although this standard applies to all groups, for White counselors it may mean that they understand how they may have directly or indirectly benefited from individual, institutional, and cultural racism as outlined in White identity development models.
    3. Culturally skilled counselors possess knowledge about their social impact on others. They are knowledgeable about communication style differences, how their style may clash with or foster the counseling process with persons of color or others different from themselves based on the A, B, and C, Dimensions, and how to anticipate the impact it may have on others.

Figure 7.2 *continued*

C. Skills
    1. Culturally skilled counselors seek out educational, consultative, and training experiences to improve their understanding and effectiveness in working with culturally different populations. Being able to recognize the limits of their competencies, they (a) seek consultation, (b) seek further training or education, (c) refer out to more qualified individuals or resources, or (d) engage in a combination of these.
    2. Culturally skilled counselors are constantly seeking to understand themselves as racial and cultural beings and are actively seeking a nonracist identity.

II. Counselor Awareness of Client's Worldview
  A. Attitudes and Beliefs
    1. Culturally skilled counselors are aware of their negative and positive emotional reactions toward other racial and ethnic groups that may prove detrimental to the counseling relationship. They are willing to contrast their own beliefs and attitudes with those of their culturally different clients in a nonjudgmental fashion.
    2. Culturally skilled counselors are aware of their stereotypes and preconceived notions that they may hold toward other racial and ethnic minority groups.

  B. Knowledge
    1. Culturally skilled counselors possess specific knowledge and information about the particular group with which they are working. They are aware of the life experiences, cultural heritage, and historical background of their culturally different clients. This particular competency is strongly linked to the "minority identity development models" available in the literature.
    2. Culturally skilled counselors understand how race, culture, ethnicity, and so forth may affect personality formation, vocational choices, manifestation of psychological disorders, help-seeking behavior, and the appropriateness or inappropriateness of counseling approaches.
    3. Culturally skilled counselors understand and have knowledge about sociopolitical influences that impinge upon the life of racial and ethnic minorities. Immigration issues, poverty, racism, stereotyping, and powerlessness may impact self esteem and self concept in the counseling process.

  C. Skills
    1. Culturally skilled counselors should familiarize themselves with relevant research and the latest findings regarding mental health and mental disorders of various ethnic and racial groups. They should actively seek out educational experiences that enrich their knowledge, understanding, and cross-cultural skills for more effective counseling behavior.
    2. Culturally skilled counselors become actively involved with minority individuals outside the counseling setting (e.g., community events, social and political functions, celebrations, friendships, neighborhood groups, and so forth) so that their perspective of minorities is more than an academic or helping exercise.

III. Culturally Appropriate Intervention Strategies
  A. Beliefs and Attitudes
    1. Culturally skilled counselors respect clients' religious and/or spiritual beliefs and values, including attributions and taboos, because they affect worldview, psychosocial functioning, and expressions of distress.
    2. Culturally skilled counselors respect indigenous helping practices and respect help-giving networks among communities of color.

continued

Figure 7.2 *continued*

3. Culturally skilled counselors value bilingualism and do not view another language as an impediment to counseling (monolingualism may be the culprit).

B. Knowledge
1. Culturally skilled counselors have a clear and explicit knowledge and understanding of the generic characteristics of counseling and therapy (culture bound, class bound, and monolingual) and how they may clash with the cultural values of various cultural groups.
2. Culturally skilled counselors are aware of institutional barriers that prevent minorities from using mental health services.
3. Culturally skilled counselors have knowledge of the potential bias in assessment instruments and use procedures and interpret findings in a way that recognizes the cultural and linguistic characteristics of the clients.
4. Culturally skilled counselors have knowledge of minority family structures, hierarchies, values, and beliefs from various cultural perspectives. They are knowledgeable about the community where a particular cultural group may reside and the resources in the community.
5. Culturally skilled counselors should be aware of relevant discriminatory practices at the social and community level that may be affecting the psychological welfare of the population being served.

C. Skills
1. Culturally skilled counselors are able to engage in a variety of verbal and nonverbal helping responses. They are able to send and receive both verbal and non-verbal messages accurately and appropriately. They are not tied down to only one method or approach to helping, but recognize that helping styles and approaches may be culture bound. When they sense that their helping style is limited and potentially inappropriate, they can anticipate and modify it.
2. Culturally skilled counselors are able to exercise institutional intervention skills on behalf of their clients. They can help clients determine whether a "problem" stems from racism or bias in others (the concept of health paranoia) so that clients do not inappropriately personalize problems.
3. Culturally skilled counselors are not averse to seeking consultation with traditional healers or religious and spiritual leaders and practitioners in the treatment of culturally different clients when appropriate.
4. Culturally skilled counselors take responsibility for interacting in the language requested by the client and, if not feasible, make appropriate referrals. A serious problem arises when the linguistic skills of a counselor do not match the language of the client. This being the case, counselors should (a) seek a translator with cultural knowledge and appropriate professional background or (b) refer to a knowledgeable and competent bilingual counselor.
5. Culturally skilled counselors have training and expertise in the use of traditional assessment and testing instruments. They not only understand the technical aspects of the instruments but are also aware of the cultural limitations. This allows them to use test instruments for the welfare of different clients.
6. Culturally skilled counselors should attend to as well as work to eliminate biases, prejudices, and discriminatory contexts in conducting evaluations and providing interventions and should develop sensitivity to issues of oppression, sexism, heterosexism, elitism, and racism.
7. Culturally skilled counselors take responsibility for educating their clients to the processes of psychological intervention, such as goals, expectations, legal rights, and the counselor's orientation.

From: Arredondo et al., 1996, pp. 57–73

INTEGRATING PERSONAL COUNSELING AND CAREER COUNSELING

Even among counseling professionals, there is a great deal of confusion as to what career counselors actually do. Consider the following scenario.

Skye is starting her third week as a career counselor in a college counseling center. She loves her job so far and thinks that career counseling seems to be her ideal counseling focus. To see clients who come in voluntarily and to focus on positive, happy things like the future is definitely the right way to go in her eyes. Skye is relieved to find that she doesn't have to use all that depressing information about mental disorders that she studied in her psychopathology class in graduate school. She thinks, "This job is going to be fun and not hard at all."

However, when Skye returns from lunch, on first day of her fourth week, a client responds to her question "How can I help you, today?" by bursting into tears. The client says, "I don't really think anyone can help me. I just want to die."

Contrary to what some believe, career counseling *is* counseling, not simply the relaying of information to clients. In fact, one of the first competency areas required by NCDA, as listed in Figure 7.1 above is individual and group counseling skills (NCDA, 1997). As the Skye scenario above indicates, there are some who believe that career counseling involves the simple relaying of career information, requires little skill, and can be accomplished in three or fewer sessions. On the other side of the coin, there are others who believe that they are unqualified to do career counseling, because their area of expertise is "personal" counseling and because there are so many more complicated additional skills involved in career counseling. The underlying and erroneous assumption being made by both these groups is the notion that people's counseling issues are separated into two distinct categories— personal issues and career issues (Herr, 1989; Blustein, 1987). There are few people who actually make this kind of distinction in their lives. People who place little importance on the work they do outside of the home still find that work and personal issues become intertwined. For example, when a client is delayed getting to a part-time job on time because of a day care problem or a client is called out of town by a supervisor at the last minute and must miss an important family function, personal and professional issues become intermingled. The more complicated one's personal and/or career roles happen to be, the more the issues become intermingled, and the harder it is for clients and counselors to sort out personal and career issues from one another. "Thus, it may be more appropriate to view career counseling as a type of psychological intervention that, at times, throughout the course of counseling, may require the counselor and client to focus on non-career concerns" (p. 225). Because of this dilemma, a number of authors have advocated that career counselors should acquire mental health skills, including an understanding of psychopathology and the effects of psychotropic drugs (Niles & Pate, 1989) and that those who practice "personal" counseling should increase their career counseling skills (Evans & Larrabee, 2002; Evans, Rotter & Gold, 2001).

The importance of integrating career counseling and personal counseling is especially significant when one considers cultural variables. As has been discussed throughout this book, counseling clients outside their reference groups leaves wide gaps in treatment. To be multiculturally competent, counselors must not separate career counseling from personal counseling. In fact, the opposite is necessary; counselors must consider the personal contexts of culturally different clients to fully succeed during the career counseling process. The next section of this chapter will begin to address the integration of career counseling skills and personal, multicultural counseling skills by integrating the NCDA and AMCD competencies.

MULTICULTURAL APPLICATIONS OF THE CAREER COUNSELING COMPETENCIES

While the NCDA competencies offer some provision for career counseling skills needed to work with culturally different populations, they fall short of the AMCD competencies in that regard. The two sets of competencies, therefore, have been integrated in the following paragraphs; they are organized by the NCDA competencies listed in Figure 7.1.

The integration of the competencies will reveal that multicultural competence in career counseling requires a number of skills, vigilance in overcoming counselor bias, awareness, and knowledge of client cultures, and a specialized knowledge of career resources.

1. "Establish and maintain productive personal relationships with individuals."

Culturally adept career counselors are able to establish trusting relationships to help clients feel at ease during the counseling process. Counselors should already have worked on their own biases and should be aware of the various ways culturally different clients may react to them. In addition, counselors should understand and be respectful of their culturally different clients by accepting their clients' worldviews (Arredondo et al., 1996). Standard approaches to rapport building may not be appropriate for all people of color, women, gays, lesbians, bisexuals, transgendered (GLBT) persons, and people with disabilities. Therefore, multiculturally competent counselors should make adjustments in their rapport building to accommodate individual client needs.

2. "Establish and maintain a productive group environment."

To maintain a culturally sensitive group, culturally competent counselors take care to choose members of the group to maximize the benefits of group counseling and minimize conflicts. Counselors accomplish this task by facilitating cultural understanding among group members, encouraging support of members, supplying resources that represent diverse groups, and promoting respect for alternative decision-making processes.

3. "Collaborate with clients in identifying personal goals."

Goal setting in career counseling has traditionally been approached as an individual process. Multiculturally competent counselors, however, should be aware that in some collectivist cultures (such as Latino/a and Native American), goals are less likely to be personal than communal (Flores & Heppner, 2002). In such cases, the inclusion of family and other community members who have a stake in the decision-making process may be important (Hawks & Muha, 1991). Counselors should understand cultural hierarchies and taboos and how those may impact client goal setting.

4. "Identify and select techniques appropriate to client or group goals, as well as to client needs, psychological states, and developmental tasks."

As mentioned earlier, not all techniques based on career counseling theories work well with all clients. Multicultural career counselors should choose techniques that best fit their clients' problems and cultural backgrounds. Adapting in this manner requires knowledge of and versatility with both career theories and counseling skill theories alike. Counselors should have sufficient knowledge of counseling theory such that if one theory clashes with a client's culture, the counselor should be able to switch to a more appropriate theoretical orientation. Counselors should understand that indigenous healing practices (such as folk remedies) may be the best approaches with some clients.

5. "Identify and understand clients' personal characteristics related to career."

Career counselors should understand that personality and personal characteristics are influenced by race, ethnicity, gender, sexual orientation, and ability status, and that these characteristics must be assessed accurately. Therefore, client characteristics must be measured by unbiased tests. If unbiased assessments are not available, multiculturally competent career counselors must be careful when interpreting biased tests for their culturally different clients.

6. "Identify and understand social contextual conditions affecting clients' careers."

Multiculturally competent career counselors should be politically aware and understand that clients are impacted by societal and institutional policies. They need not only to understand client feelings of powerlessness and internalized oppression, but also to recognize the important contributions made by oppressed individuals (such as immigrant workers, low-paid factory workers, and retail employees).

7. "Identify and understand familial, subcultural, and cultural structures as they are related to clients' careers."

Multiculturally competent career counselors should understand the expectations that families and cultural structures place on clients in their work environments. Counselors not only need to understand, but also respect how the family hierarchy, and cultural values and expectations impact decision making.

8. "Identify and understand clients' career decision-making processes."

The multiculturally competent career counselor should be aware that each client is different, and that acculturation will dictate the need for family members and/or other important members of the community to become involved in the process. Counselors should be careful not to impose their own decision-making strategies onto the client or to expect that client decision-making styles will be completely dictated by their cultural groups.

9. "Identify and understand clients' attitudes toward work and workers."
10. "Identify and understand clients' biases toward work and workers based on gender, race, and cultural stereotypes."

Multicultural career counselors realize that it is especially important to assess culturally different clients' beliefs and attitudes toward white (or majority) workers and toward the organization for which they work. In addition, counselors should be aware of how race, culture, ethnicity, gender, sexual orientation, and minority status affect the client's vocational choices, taking into account the effects of immigration, poverty (welfare), individual discrimination, stereotyping, and institutional discrimination.

11. "Challenge and encourage clients to take action to prepare for and initiate role transitions by locating sources of relevant information and experience, and obtaining and interpreting information and experiences and acquiring skills needed to make role transitions."

Multiculturally competent career counselors understand how poverty, discrimination, racism, and so forth limit client access to information, inhibit client ability to take action, and limit the scope of possibilities clients may see for themselves.

12. "Assist the client to acquire a set of employability and job search skills."

Culturally competent career counselors must be aware of discriminatory practices at social and community agencies that may affect the psychological welfare of the client. Also counselors must be aware of their own biases (especially middle-class values) because these biases may color their ability to empathize with and assist clients in their job search.

13. "Support and challenge clients to examine life-work roles, including the balance of work, leisure, family, and community in their careers."

Balancing work and family is a challenge for all clients and becomes an especially difficult challenge when they are working for minimum wage and raising a family at the same time. Multiculturally competent career counselors must realize that clients may need to be assisted in finding time for leisure and community to balance their busy lives.

Counseling Culturally Diverse Children

Another commonly held misconception about career counseling, even among counselors, is that career counseling is only for adults or adolescents in high school who are deciding between college and work. Consider the following scenario.

Michael is beginning his first school counseling practicum in an elementary school. His practicum instructor has required him to run two groups, one of which has to be a career development group. Richard relays this information to his site supervisor, Ms. Cooper, who told him this requirement is ridiculous and says that the only career development activity she does routinely is the annual career fair.

The fact is that career development is a cradle to the grave process. Individuals benefit from career counseling at any age. In fact, members of oppressed groups tend to limit their career choices very early in life because of misinformation and stereotypes (Gottfredson, 1981). It is crucial, therefore, that career counseling begin as early as possible in the lives of culturally different clients. The American School Counselor Association (ASCA) (2002) recommends career development activities in the elementary school in its National Model, and the National Career Development Guidelines Framework (ACRN) describes goals and indicators for school children from elementary to high school grades. Many of the skills described in this chapter are useful for school counselors when they work with children and parents from racially and culturally different groups.

STAGES OF CAREER COUNSELING

When counselors master the integration of career and multicultural competencies, the career counseling in action becomes much more effective and relevant for clients from culturally different groups. All counseling proceeds through various stages, and counselors-in-training need to become familiar with these stages to assure that their clients make steady progress through each stage. The stages of career counseling are similar to and different from the stages of other types of counseling. Niles and Harris-Bowlsbey (2005) divide career counseling into three phases: the initial phase (in which a working alliance is established); the middle phase or working phase (in which goals are set and reset); and the ending or termination stage. Other authors have developed more elaborate career counseling stages. For example, Yost and Corbishley (1987) divided career counseling into eight different stages: Stage 1 (Initial Assessment), Stage 2 (Self-Understanding), Stage 3 (Making Sense of Self-Understanding Data), Stage 4 (Generating Alternatives), Stage 5 (Obtaining Occupational Information), Stage 6 (Making Choices), Stage 7 (Making Plans), and Stage 8 (Implementing Plans).

In this section, the eight stages of the Yost and Corbishley model will be outlined in more detail, and the integrated NCDA/AMCD multicultural career competencies will be discussed within this framework, utilizing an ongoing case study for further illumination of the multicultural career counseling process. The case study begins with some background on the client, Luis Alverez, and his career counselor, Ivy:

Luis Alverez is a twenty-six-year-old Puerto Rican man living an openly gay lifestyle in a large city in the Southeast. He is tall, attractive, outgoing, and energetic. Luis is appropriately dressed for his interview and appears physically and intellectually strong. While Luis is openly gay in the city where he lives, he has yet to come out to his family, who live in New York City. Luis is a high school graduate who grew up in poverty. After graduating from high school, he accompanied a couple of friends on a road trip to Florida and never went back to New York. Currently, he is employed as an Assistant Manager at a national chain of fast food restaurants where he has worked for the past five years. It is a job he has come to despise. Luis is undecided between becoming a chef or an interior designer. He jokingly states that interior design is just too clichéd for a gay man. However, he wants to decide now, because he believes that his life is going nowhere fast.

Luis has strong ties to the gay community but also has strong familial ties and deep appreciation of his Puerto Rican heritage. Unfortunately, he says, he has suffered discrimination and lack of tolerance under both identities.

Luis has been assigned to Ivy, who is a forty-two-year-old career counselor with seventeen years of counseling experience. Ivy is African American (born and raised in the southeastern United States) and heterosexual. Therefore, her work with Luis will involve a number of cross-cultural dimensions—gender, race, ethnicity, culture, geography, age, sexual orientation, and socioeconomic status.

Stage I, Initial Assessment: Part I, Establishing the Counseling Relationship

In this initial phase of the Yost and Corbishley model, the career counselor prepares for the counseling relationship, meets and greets the client, establishes rapport and relationship with the client, and creates a structure for the career counseling process. This beginning stage is always important, but it is even more essential to establish the counseling relationship effectively in cases of cross-cultural counselor/client dyads (client and counselor from two different cultural groups) than in cases of same-culture dyads. Because stereotypes, discrimination, and bias are commonplace in U.S. society, it is not uncommon for diverse clients to mistrust and harbor suspicion about counseling. These attitudes can easily sabotage the counselor-client relationship if it is not established effectively from the start (Whaley, 2001).

Counselor Preparation

The first step in establishing the counseling relationship in a multicultural career counseling situation is counselor preparation, especially counselor introspection, in which counselors assess their own biases and stereotypes (Gold et al., 2002; Ridley et al., 1998). If the counselor is aware of any possibility of harm coming to a client because of the counselor's own prejudices, then the client should be referred to a different counselor while the initial counselor works on these issues. More importantly, while effective counselors know themselves better than anyone else, they still may have blinders on regarding certain issues. It is always good practice for counselors to engage in ongoing supervision with someone who may offer an objective opinion of their work.

In previous chapters, we discussed cultural mistrust on the part of clients from culturally different groups, client views of counselors from the dominant European American cultural group, and client reactions to institutional racism. When preparing for the first contact, it is helpful for the counselor to understand the possibility that the client may have negative perceptions not only of the counseling process, but also of the counselor (Helms & Cook, 1999; Ridley, 1995; Whaley, 2001). The counselor should plan to be as open and honest with the client as possible and understand the origins of client feelings of anger and distrust.

While counselors cannot predict specific client reactions, they need to employ strategies to facilitate the growth of good client-counselor working relationships. Regardless of cultural background, some clients are easier to relate to than others, but it is the responsibility of counselors to establish strong working alliances. Such an alliance can transcend racial, cultural, gender, sexual orientation, and other differences, as the continuing case study demonstrates:

Ivy explores the values she holds as an African American woman, careful to consider the ones that may interfere with her acceptance of her client, Luis. Ivy's experiences with gay males have been limited to friends, who were treated as "mascots" among her circle of female friends. They were never full members of the group. Ivy realizes now how patronizing that behavior was and decides that she must monitor any maternal or protective feelings she may have toward Luis. She will make sure to solicit her supervisor's help on this.

Ivy also has been taught by family to be suspicious of Puerto Ricans and other Latinos or Latinas. In the past, the reasons for this suspicion were never clear, but today she believes it comes from the fact that Latinas and Latinos now outnumber African

Americans as the largest ethnic minority group in the United States. Ivy thinks that her family and friends are fearful that African Americans may lose their privileged status among oppressed groups. Ivy has also never knowingly resented Latinos or Latinas, but she is aware that it is difficult to dismiss what has been learned over a long period of time. She will inform her supervisor of this issue as well.

Ivy has counseled her share of male clients, but she believes that this client will expect to explore his masculinity in more depth than other clients have, since he brings up that issue in relation to his sexual orientation. Her familiarity with gender socialization among Latinas and Latinos will be helpful here.

Although her middle-class upbringing may have dictated certain values about school and career, Ivy has never had problems accepting people from all socioeconomic backgrounds. She has been successful with very poor and very affluent clients, and she does not foresee a problem with Luis in this regard.

Meeting and Greeting

Meeting anyone for the first time can be awkward. The awkwardness of meeting a new client may be slight for the counselor, but it may be nerve-wracking for the client. Although career counseling may seem less stigmatizing than other kinds of counseling, clients may feel just as vulnerable nonetheless. Members of some cultures frown upon seeking help outside of the family, even if it is career help rather than psychological help. Therefore, some clients will be reluctant and nervous about entering into any kind of counseling. The counselor must make the client feel as comfortable as possible the first time the client walks into the counseling agency.

To facilitate client comfort, the physical environment of the counseling agency needs to be as welcoming as the agency can afford. For example, if certain cultural groups are especially likely to be clients at the agency, the agency should provide waiting room magazines representative of those cultural groups. If subscriptions are not in the budget, counselors may be able to obtain copies of magazines from other sources, including fellow counselors at the agency. When clients see familiar magazines and books, the message to clients is that they belong there. Also, if possible, pictures of community members and the staff taken at specific community events (festivals, block parties, holiday celebrations, and so forth) should be hung on the walls, because this reinforces the image that the agency is part of the community and further helps clients to feel welcome.

The employment of individuals from underrepresented groups in the front office also signals that the agency is an accepting and welcoming environment for all. Ideally, bilingual staff members will be available to accommodate clients who are more comfortable speaking in their first language. Notices and printed materials should be available in more than one language, and any pictures of people on the wall should illustrate a diverse population. These cosmetic details increase the possibility that counselors will establish rapport with culturally different clients and that the clients will return to the agency after their initial meetings.

Greeting clients for the first time can also affect rapport. Job search literature states that job interviewers and interviewees have twenty-five seconds to make a first impression. This is true in counselor-client relationships as well. In the 1980s and 1990s, much was written about the appropriate way to address a culturally different client. For instance, some authors suggested that African Americans clients felt inferior and disrespected when white counselors called them by their first names (reminiscent of slavery and service jobs) (Sue & Sue, 2003). Perhaps the best advice to consider when addressing all clients is to address them by their title and last name (Mr. Alverez) and to wait until clients give permission to use their first names. Counselors should not ask for that permission. Once clients get to know their counselors better, they may invite their counselors to call them by the name their friends and family use.

Similarly, many clients may believe that using the counselor's first name diminishes the counselor's credibility (Sue & Sue, 2003). The hierarchical nature of many cultures demands that the counselor (someone with knowledge and wisdom) be treated with respect. For example, early in my career, an African American woman client discovered after our second session that I had a Ph.D. She was embarrassed for calling me Miss Evans and apologized profusely. Even though I told her it did not matter to me, it mattered to her that she was disrespectful of my position and me. During our time together, our relationship grew strong, and she accomplished a great deal in therapy. We never were on a first-name basis, however. I was always Dr. Evans to her and she was always Mrs. Jones to me.

The counselor must appear competent, confident, and in control (but not controlling or arrogant) during these first minutes. Herr, Cramer, and Niles (2004) also point out that self-disclosure on the part of the counselor, an attitude of noncondemnation toward the client, and an aura of wisdom and stability on the part of the counselor are important qualities to bring across during the first meeting with the client. However clients are greeted, counselors should exude warmth and understanding.

Rapport and Relationship Building

The foundation of counseling is the counselor-client relationship, and there is no relationship if there is no rapport. The relationship between culturally different clients and counselors is especially important (Bingham & Ward, 1994; Constantine, 1998; Flores et al., 2003). The skills important for rapport building with culturally different clients are taught to every beginning-level counselor, and include such skills as reflection of feelings, open rather than yes or no questions, paraphrasing, and summarizing (Niles & Harris-Bowlsbey, 2005; Brammer, 1993). More importantly, genuineness, respect, and empathy create an environment of warmth and caring for all clients, including those from different cultural backgrounds (Patterson, 1996; Pedersen, 1996).

Counselors of culturally diverse clients are faced with a greater challenge establishing credibility than counselors working with clients of the same background as themselves, but overcoming the challenges is essential for a good working relationship (Ridley et al., 1998; Sue & Sue, 2003). Credibility is enhanced not only by counselors discussing their credentials, but also by their apparent genuine interest and openness to client questions. Also, counselor self-disclosure helps establish trustworthiness and genuineness (Ivy, D'Andrea, Ivy & Simek-Morgan, 2002).

Career counseling research reports that many ethnic minority clients prefer direct answers to their direct questions (Sue & Sue, 2003). This type of communication is not uncommon in career counseling, and it may be essential in building rapport with ethnic minority clients. However, it is important not to use research data to stereotype individual clients. Every client is unique no matter his or her cultural or racial background. While it is important to be knowledgeable about cultural influences on career development, it is equally important to realize that a client is an individual within the context of his or her culture. Along those same lines, the culture of counseling promotes skills such as genuineness and empathy to build rapport and establish relationships with clients. However, counselors must adapt those skills to the needs of the individual client. As such, Pedersen (1996) warns that "respect for client, genuineness, and empathic understanding are themselves products of a cultural context, and they will need to be interpreted differently in each complex and dynamic cultural situation" (p. 236).

To reduce time spent gathering data in the initial session, some agencies ask clients to fill out an intake form, which can be as simple or as complicated as the agency desires. The form should be available in the predominant languages of clients served by the agency. While many intake forms collect only basic client demographic data and a brief description of the client's problem, some intake forms are a great deal more in-depth and may include such information as work history, family work history, history of mental and physical health problems, illegal drug history, current family situation, and so forth (Yost & Coblishley, 1984). If the client fills out an intake form, the counselor may want to take the liberty of following up on some of the client's answers during the rapport building stage, for example saying to the client, "I see that you play soccer, tell me a little more about this activity." Or the counselor may highlight items that the counselor may have in common with the client, for instance, "My very first job in high school was with your fast food chain. Tell me how you got started there." Connecting in this way with the client enables the client to relax. However, counselors also need to balance connecting with the client and overemphasizing similarities. Highlighting one or two similarities to get the client talking is advisable, but counselors should be aware that an overemphasis on similarities may appear to the client as if the counselor is trying too hard to find common ground where none really exists (Brown & Brooks, 1991). Many oppressed groups (ethnic minorities as well as GLBT persons, and people with disabilities) value their uniqueness and emphasizing similarities tends to minimize that uniqueness.

Another rapport-building strategy is to mention racial and cultural dissimilarities with the client early in the first session (Brown & Brooks, 1991). Dealing with racial and cultural differences early in the relationship rather than waiting until it is obvious that the client is having difficulty with these differences is advisable. Such an approach clears the air and may prevent culturally different clients from prematurely terminating counseling. The counselor might introduce the topic by saying something like this:

"Mr. Alverez (notice that the counselor addresses the client by his last name), *we have clients from many backgrounds come to our center. Sometimes clients and counselors of different races, like us, are paired up in the initial interview, and these pairings have worked out very well. However, we want our clients to feel comfortable with their counselors. Because counseling is so personal, we believe you should be matched with someone*

who is most likely to meet your needs. Often clients prefer to work with counselors of their own racial/cultural group or similar sexual orientation. We try our best to accommodate them. If you would like to be paired with a counselor from your own racial group or sexual orientation, I will try to arrange it. If you do decide to stay with me, I feel confident that I will be able to help you with your problem, and we can discuss any racial/sexual orientation issues that might arise as we go along."

Introducing cultural differences in this manner gives the client an "out" that he or she can live with, and it brings race and cultural issues to the forefront. However, keep in mind that the opposite may be true in the case of European American clients working with a counselor of color. For example, an African American counselor stated in a workshop I attended that when she brought up race with her white clients, the subject seemed to make them uncomfortable, nervous, or defensive. She decided that in the future if a client reacted in this way, she would quickly add, "You don't have to make up your mind today. If you want, you can go home and think about it. Even if you decide to stay with me, if at any time you feel uncomfortable about working with me because of racial or cultural differences, you are welcome to ask to be transferred to another counselor and you won't have to clear it through me first." A statement such as this may lower client discomfort and may enhance relationship building. In addition, some agencies include a question about counselor preferences on the intake form. In fact, it is usually easier on both the client and the counselor if such preferences are handled through the intake form in order to avoid uncomfortable face-to-face situations. Then, if no counselors are available who match the client's preferred list of background characteristics, the assigned counselor is able to address this issue in session. Depending on the client's racial identity status, it may be necessary in some cases to refer the client to another counseling agency if the client is adamant about counselor preference.

Relationship building may also be enhanced when counselors make clients aware that they are familiar with their culture (Brown & Brooks, 1991). One caveat applies here: It is better to be modest about cultural knowledge than to show off. Instead of going on at length about their cultural knowledge, counselors should let the clients do most of the talking about their culture. Counselors should gain knowledge about culture to educate themselves to be better prepared to assist with the cultural issues clients bring to counseling, not to impress their clients. The ongoing case study illustrates how the counselor can subtly introduce her knowledge of the client's culture into the discussion in order to build rapport:

Ivy says, "Mr. Alverez, I have visited Puerto Rico a couple of times and have enjoyed my visits. I have tried to learn as much as I can about Puerto Rico and about the culture through these visits and through my friends. My spoken Spanish is awful, but I understand more than I can speak. I'm hoping that what I know of your culture will be helpful in our work together. I hope, too, that you will let me know when I've got it all wrong."

Creating Structure

Some counselors tend to overlook the essential relationship-building task of providing a structure to the counseling process. The more the counselor can tell the client about what will happen during the counseling process, the more comfortable clients will feel about that process, and the more receptive they will be toward counseling. In addition to easing client worries about the counseling process, structuring helps build counselor credibility by demonstrating the counselor's professionalism (Sue & Sue, 2003). Structuring includes informing clients of the procedures that will be followed, explaining the rules of confidentiality, defining the limitations of the counseling process, discussing any limitations on the issues that can be addressed and the possible outcomes, and relating rules about attendance, tardiness, and fees. Counselors should also explain to clients how counseling sessions work without using jargon or complicated terms (Niles & Harris-Bowlsbey, 2005), as illustrated in the ongoing case study. Ivy introduces structure to the session by saying:

"Mr. Alvarez, what I thought we'd do first is to spend a little bit of our time getting to know one another and then we'll talk some about counseling—what it is, how it's done, what your role is, and what my role is. Then if everything sounds okay to you, we'll go on and talk about what brought you in to see me—what the problem seems to be. How does that sound to you?"

After roles are discussed, Ivy discloses her career counseling theory as illustrated below. Whichever way the counselor chooses to explain the counseling process, the outcome should be that the client feels both informed and comfortable about what is to come:

I believe that it is important that all clients find careers that are compatible with their personalities. Through counseling, I can help them take a good look at their own personalities to see whether or not the career they are interested in gives them an opportunity to use their greatest personality strengths. I believe that clients are unhappy and dissatisfied with their work when they haven't found careers that match their personalities.

For some clients, confidentiality is one of the most important features of the structuring process. For instance, many ethnic minority populations frown upon sharing family problems outside the family and so confidentiality helps these clients feel more secure about engaging in the counseling process. Gay, lesbian, and bisexual clients many need to be assured that if they have chosen not to be out of the closet with family, friends, and/or coworkers, the counseling process will not result in their being outed. Reassurances about confidentiality may also curb clients' feelings of cultural distrust of the counselor (Brown & Brooks, 1991; Whaley, 2001; Helms & Cook, 1999).

A structuring method known as role induction also helps to reduce client anxiety, and it has been effective with ethnic minority clients whose familiarity with counseling may be limited (Galassi et al., 1992; Niles & Bowlsbey, 2005). Essentially, role induction involves informing clients of what is expected of them during the counseling process. The counselor's role is also presented. Spokane (1991) recommends that counselors create handouts that describe both the counselor's and client's responsibilities and give these handouts to clients. Some agencies provide handouts that describe what the counselor will *not* do, explaining not only the limitations of the counseling agency but also the limitations of the counseling process itself.

Once a structure is in place, the relationship-building stage should continue until the counselor perceives that the client is comfortable enough to discuss his or her problem. Counselors may find that, when working with clients from oppressed groups, rapport and relationship building may go on for several sessions. Continued rapport and relationship building is time well spent, because the counselor is able to use the additional time to regroup and approach the client more slowly to strengthen the relationship when resistance is encountered.

Whatever the case, the primary goal at the beginning of counseling is to make a connection with the client via preparation, successful meeting and greeting, rapport building, and structuring. If the client is comfortable with the process, better results can be achieved. Counselors who continue to have problems establishing relationships with culturally different clients should seek consultation or supervision from someone with a specialty in multicultural counseling. Possibly the counselor may be unconsciously communicating negative verbal and/or nonverbal messages to the client, which can be seen in a videotape or via live supervision.

Stage I, Initial Assessment: Part 2, Identifying the Counseling Issues

Once a counselor-client relationship has been firmly established, the career counseling process enters Part 2 of Stage 1, identifying the counseling issues. In this phase, the counselor must answer two questions: (1) Is there a career problem here? and (2) If there is a career problem, what kind of problem is it? Assessment of career issues begins with the first session, usually via an intake interview. Often the client's presenting career problems are not the real counseling issues. Sometimes clients think they want to change their careers, when in reality they want to see a change in the organization they work for. Or sometimes the real issue is not specific to career development. For example, in the case of a woman who wants to change careers because she has been sexually harassed on the job, but has not yet addressed the effect the harassment has had on her, an assessment of the real counseling issue is imperative for counseling to proceed. Part of the counselor's job is to determine if career counseling is appropriate, or if the client should tackle psychological or emotional issues first. Crites (1981), among others, has recommended that career counseling follow personal counseling. The rationale is that if an individual has emotional or psychological challenges, informed career decisions are not possible. Career counselors should have an open mind and must be able to assist clients whatever the issues.

Determining a client's emotional and psychological state is particularly delicate with ethnic or other minority clients who may be hesitant, nervous, or cautious about the counseling process in general (Highlen & Sudarsky-Glieser, 1996). The counselor must determine the severity of the emotional status of the client through psychological training and knowledge of the client's culture. Counselors must be careful not to use European American standards of mental health to evaluate people of color (Ridley, 1995). So, too they must be careful not to apply sexist or heterosexist standards to women or to GLBT individuals. The combination of knowledge of psychiatric disorders and cultural manifestations of those disorders is paramount when serving diverse populations appropriately. If a counselor discovers that the client's emotional and mental health issues may interfere with career decision-making processes, this determination should be discussed with the client before proceeding.

Ridley, Li, and Hill (1998) have constructed a culturally sensitive model for assessing culturally diverse clients, outlining several decision points that occur during assessment. First, counselors must decide whether or not they possess sufficient information to make decisions. The counselor may need to collect more data from the client or other sources (such as family, spouse, standardized tests). Next, the counselor needs to decide which data are influenced by culture and which are idiosyncratic to that individual. Counselors use baseline information about various cultures gathered from the literature and other reliable sources (such as National Institute of Health, U.S. Department of Labor) to make this determination. If the client's behavior is outside of the baseline for his or her culture, the counselor may hypothesize that the behavior is likely to be idiosyncratic and set about trying to prove or disprove the hypothesis. The counselor may look for environmental influences to explain the behavior (such as hostile work environment, neighborhood environment, domestic violence issues). If the hypothesis still holds, most likely the client needs to work on his or her psychological issues before proceeding to career counseling. Whether or not the client's issue is strictly career-related, counselors should have the expertise to work on that issue. If counselors do not have this expertise, the client should be referred to a more appropriate counselor (such as a psychotherapist) and asked to return for career counseling when the psychological problem has been satisfactorily addressed.

If there are no intervening psychological issues, the next decision is to determine the type of career counseling needed. Campbell and Cellini (1981) have identified over thirty-seven different career problems in their diagnostic taxonomy. These problems are divided into four categories: (a) problems in decision making, (b) problems in implementing career plans, (c) problems in organization/institutional performance, and (d) problems in organizational/institutional adaptation. Some specific client issues that would fall under these categories include performance anxiety, depression over failures, and role confusion (Lowman, 1993). Each of the problems listed by Campbell and Cellini can be exacerbated by discrimination and bias. For example, in a situation where a client is seen as deficient by a supervisor who holds culturally different supervisees to a higher standard, the client's problems may be the result of racism, sexism, or heterosexism. Counselors must discuss client issues with their clients in enough detail to ascertain exactly what the career problems are, while keeping in mind that these problems may be negatively influenced by larger social/cultural barriers.

Stage 2, Self-Understanding

Once particular career counseling issues are identified, career counselors need to assist clients in becoming more aware of their personal interests, abilities, values, and personalities (Krumboltz & Coon, 1995). To expedite this process, interests, abilities, values, and personality are typically measured through standardized testing. However, with diverse clients, culture and ethnicity heavily influence these personal factors, and therefore both Ridley and colleagues (1998) and Highlen and Sudarsky-Gleiser (1994) recommend nonstandardized assessment for culturally different clients. This is because, as discussed in Chapter 6, standardized testing has come under great criticism for its bias against ethnic minorities, so it is best to be very careful and knowledgeable when using standardized testing with culturally different clients. In addition to nonstandardized testing, qualitative interviewing allows counselors to obtain more information on clients' cultural characteristics. Assisting clients to develop an awareness of their cultures and to internalize this information is essential in multicultural career counseling. For example, an African American sixth grade boy decides to stop studying because his peers tell him he is trying to be white. Through cultural self-awareness exploration during the counseling process, he may learn about his cultural identity and the importance of education in the history of African Americans. An Asian woman works with a group of strong European women and is uncomfortable with her job setting because the women disrespect their elders and their spouses. She may discover through exploration of her own culture during the career counseling process how to become tolerant to different world views. Similarly, the friends and family of a twenty-two-year-old Latina have teased her about her interest in becoming a veterinarian, to the point that she has chosen a sociology major. Through cultural self-awareness exploration during counseling, she may learn to broaden her concept of *familismo* to include seeking their support to pursue a career they may not have chosen for her. And as a final example, a gay adolescent male who has become a moody, withdrawn adolescent due to discrimination based on his sexual orientation may learn through self-awareness exploration during counseling how to cope with discrimination.

Expanding on the above examples, the following three sections will explore in further detail how cultural issues, sociopolitical influences, and client attitudes and biases toward work and other workers affect client self-awareness and understanding. Counselors who understand these factors in depth will be able to help clients obtain the self-awareness and understanding they need to obtain during this third stage of the career counseling process, and move on to subsequent stages of the process.

Cultural Issues

Arredondo and colleagues (1996) state that knowledge of a group's cultural heritage, including its history, religion, language, and family structures, is important information for the culturally skilled counselor. However, simply being knowledgeable about this information is not enough. Counselors still need to understand how all of these factors influence their clients. To gain that fuller understanding, counselors should collect not just the cultural facts from the client, but also ascertain their clients' perception of their cultures, unearth their clients' cultural and racial identity statuses, and then explore the socio-political barriers their clients have experienced (personally or vicariously through the experiences of others within their cultures). Counselors may assess this information by interviewing the client using the Career-in-Culture Interview protocol, which includes getting the client's career story, having the client appraise his or her skills, and an exploration into the client's cultural background, values, and family expectations, the client's view of his or her own community, and experiences with or beliefs about oppression and barriers (Ponterotto, Rivera, & Sueyoshi, 2000). Highlen and Sudarsky-Gleiser (1996) suggest obtaining this information via storytelling, art, discussion, meditation, and dream analysis. These methods all provide the counselor with an opportunity to open a discussion of cultural issues with a client. Highlen & Sudarsky-Gleiser also advocate asking qualitative questions in order to assess the career characteristics of clients. For example, they suggest asking, "What activities do you participate in where you lose track of time?" (p. 323) in order to ascertain a client's vocational calling. In fact, if counselors wish to forgo formal testing, they can access a great deal of information by just asking the client qualitative questions such as

- "I learn more about people when I know more about their stories. Tell me the story of your life as a(n) _____" (fills in client's cultural/racial group).
- "Have you ever been discriminated against? If so what were the circumstances? How do you think _____ (racism, sexism, classism, heterosexism, ableism) affects you now? How do you think it will affect you in the future?"
- "Tell me a little about how you are the same or different from people in your culture or your family."
- "How would the head of your family describe you?"

The counselor must be sensitive to any information learned that may prove detrimental to a client's career development, such as acculturative stress, conflicts clients may have with their family and cultural group regarding differences in acculturation, feelings of not fitting into any cultural group, racial identity problems, and so forth. These may be issues that need to be worked out in advance to best facilitate moving into more action-oriented stages of the career counseling process. Depending on the client's cultural group and level of acculturation within that cultural group, the counselor may suggest individual or group counseling to approach these issues.

Several studies have found that while ethnic minorities have encountered and identified barriers to entering their chosen professions, they have been able to succeed because of support from family and friends (McWhirter et al., 1998). The implication is that with support from the right people, barriers are easier to overcome. Lee (1984) has found in a comparative study of adolescents that parental impact on career decisions is greater for minority children than it is for white children. Therefore, the counselors must always assess family influences on their clients. In fact, when counseling people from collectivist cultures (Latinos and Latinas, American Indian) counselors should consider inviting their clients' families into the counseling process when possible to give input into counseling, since clients from these cultures may be unwilling to make career decisions without family input (Fernandez, 1988). However, this may prove difficult in some situations, as it is in the case of Luis, who, though a member of a collectivist culture, is also gay in a culture whose members of the group often disapprove of his sexual orientation:

Luis' beliefs about his cultural group and his perceptions of what is expected of him are the focus of many of his early career counseling sessions with Ivy. There are legitimate reasons why gay, lesbian, bisexual, and transgendered individuals never disclose their sexual orientation to certain groups, and it may be that Luis will decide against such a disclosure, but first he and the counselor need to explore why he is in conflict and whether or not coming out to his family will ease that conflict. Luis may decide that there are specific members of his family that he wants to come out to because of the guilt feelings he has about lying to them. The fact that he is reluctant to choose a career that he believes will be a red flag to his sexual orientation indicates that there are members of his family that he does not ever want to know about his sexuality. Luis and Ivy discuss and explore the possible reactions of his family members and how his disclosure may affect his relationships with them. Ivy encourages Luis to read the biographies of other gay Latinos (for example, Michael Nava's chapter, "Abuelo: My Grandfather, Raymond Acuna," in A Member of the Family: Gay Men Write About Their Families, *edited and with an introduction by John Preston, Plume, 1994) to get some idea of how they successfully handled family reactions.*

Socio-political Influences

In addition to looking at personal cultural influences that may affect self-awareness and understanding in ethnic minority and other oppressed clients during the career counseling process, counselors also have to look at and integrate socio-political variables, such as racism, sexism, heterosexism, discrimination, and internalized oppression. This has been discussed in much of the career counseling literature. For instance, Hawks and Muha (1991) believe that counselors need to make sure their clients know that they are knowledgeable about racism and that they are aware that it still exists. Additionally, Helms and Piper (1994) suggest that career counselors need to become aware that a person's race or culture may be a limiting factor in obtaining and/or maintaining a career because of discrimination and other institutional barriers (such as the proverbial glass ceiling). Similarly, Krumboltz and Coon (1995) state that counselors should recognize the limitations faced by women, who typically must juggle several roles at one time. To help counter the socio-political factors diverse clients are faced with, counselors should assist clients in developing coping skills, understanding societal stereotyping of certain careers, and finding role models who defy stereotypes and who will encourage clients to broaden their career search options.

Counselors must also be aware of how sexual and racial discrimination can manifest itself as workplace harassment. Harassment can be either overt or covert. In the latter case, the subtle behaviors of individuals in the workplace many not seem to be overt sexual or racial harassment, but clients feel uncomfortable around such persons nonetheless. A client's perceptions of harassing behaviors are a legitimate concern and should be addressed during the counseling process in order to explore client self-awareness and understanding. The counselor should not minimize these perceptions but should explore how they are helping or hurting the client. If these perceptions are disturbing or hurtful, the counselor needs to outline strategies for both coping with the present situation and for changing the situation through client action.

Much of what clients need to do to deal with discrimination and harassment is covered in Chapter 8 of this book. An example of a strategy that may empower the client is to encourage the client to collect data documenting discrimination. If the client is unable to substantiate the claim, he or she may alternatively wish to learn how to cope with oppressive policies and individuals. Coping strategies that have been said to be effective include diplomatic confrontation, learning to control one's anger toward the situation through anger management, learning to come to some peace with the situation via spirituality and prayer, proving one's worth to oneself and others by excelling at one's job, garnering support by joining supportive organizations, ignoring or avoiding the perpetrator, or if all else fails, finding a new job (Evans, 1997). Luis's career issues are certainly impacted by socio-political factors, as the continuing case study illustrates:

Although Luis does not feel much discrimination from fellow co-workers where he is currently employed, he worries that to sustain a career as a chef he may need to hide his sexual orientation. It is one of the concerns he has about changing to this new career—how will he be accepted as a gay Latino? Luis is less worried about his sexual orientation regarding interior design but is concerned about whether or not he will be able to get a job in the city where he now lives—where there are few Latinos and Latinas and some very narrow-minded people regarding race and culture.

Clients from culturally different groups not only experience discrimination, but they often internalize the negative stereotypes that are part and parcel of discrimination. These internalized negative stereotypes limit clients' career development because they lower self-esteem and increase doubt in their own abilities. These kinds of beliefs are evident when girls (and boys) use their gender to explain their inability to perform certain career duties. For example, a seventh grade girl (who was a straight A math student during elementary school) justifying her C in pre-algebra because "Everybody knows girls can't do math." Counselors should assess the impact of stereotyping on clients to help them reach a state of more positive self-awareness and understanding, from which they may evaluate their worth more realistically.

Client Attitudes and Biases Toward Work and Other Workers

In addition to cultural and socio-political influences, reaching self-awareness and understanding in this stage of the career counseling process is also impacted by clients' own attitudes toward work and toward other workers.

Attitudes toward work may have a cultural origin. For example, in some ethnic minority cultures, competition is discouraged, whereas competition is valued by the dominant culture in the United States. Further, sometimes competition creates tension among individuals from culturally different groups. Counselors need to work with clients so that clients do not perceive competition as cultural warfare and therefore do not take personally any defeats or wins in the competitive arena. If the competitors are, in fact, using cultural dominance as a means to suppress the competition, then counselors need to help clients decide what is in the client's best interest in terms of dealing with the situation.

Competition is not the only factor that impacts attitudes toward work among culturally different clients. Helms and Cook (1999) point out that the policies and expectations in many places of employment reflect dominant white European American values, which may be in direct conflict with cultural experiences of some groups. Helms and Cook suggest that many ethnic minority clients' careers may be limited, because the work culture may be foreign to them. Such a client does not know what to do to fit in (Thomas & Alderfer, 1989). Additionally, women clients, those with disabilities, as well as gay, lesbian, bisexual, and transgendered clients may feel at odds with the prevailing old boy network of many workplaces, in which there exists an underlying assumption by management that able-bodied, heterosexual men are in control and women, sexual minorities, and people with disabilities are subordinate. Such attitudes may cause these clients to feel powerless and discouraged, believing that there is no chance that they will have real success in their careers. Perceptions of work, therefore, may be influenced by this perception of difference. Stereotypes about ethnic minority workers prevail. Some groups are perceived as lazy, and those stereotypes can color an employer's perceptions of that group's work styles. In fact, stereotypes such as this may lead to self-fulfilling prophesy because the client knows that co-workers or supervisors expect laziness and may decide to cut corners, since he or she will be blamed for slacking off anyway.

Although clients may have negative attitudes toward work for the reasons described above, sometimes clients' own issues impact self-awareness. Clients themselves may harbor biases and prejudices against other groups. For instance, they may complain that certain groups are taking over, or that certain groups are unclean, lazy, or stupid. Sometimes animosity is aimed toward the supervisor, whom the client may correctly or incorrectly think is prejudiced or biased. Counselors must work with clients to discover these biases, which may result in problems within the workplace and lack of success in interpersonal relationships. Again familiarity with the racial/cultural identity models and the client's cultural history will help prepare the counselor to challenge clients on their beliefs and help them to grow into self-awareness and understanding.

Stage 3, Making Sense of Self-Understanding Data

After clients have explored with their counselors the factors described above and reached a point of career self-awareness and understanding, the counselor's job is to help clients synthesize self-awareness with career objectives. Clients have to make decisions about the skills they want to use, pinpoint the activities that they are interested in, make up their minds about what values are most important to them, and reach conclusions about how well their cultural and personality traits will fit in certain occupations. Yost and Corbishley have outlined a set of factors to help counselors and clients approach this sorting out process. Through the intake interview and/or the initial assessment, as well as through appropriate standardized tests, clients discover their work preference factors, such as work tasks (routine, physical), working conditions (environment, teamwork, autonomy), location (indoor/outdoor, geographical area), and benefits (prestige, salary, challenge). Other factors outlined by Yost and Corbishley include information about clients' parents and other significant adults, and their work and attitudes about work, and their early experiences with work. Cultural influences will have been assessed so that clients are aware of these factors as well as environmental factors such as discrimination and socioeconomic status.

To put all this information together in the Yost and Corbishley system, clients are asked to prioritize the factors, using any prioritizing system that seems to work for them. The goal is for clients to come up with only five top factors important in the work they choose. Yost and Corbishley also suggest that clients list three to five factors they would want to avoid at all costs.

Clients will now have generated a list of their work-related preferences, taking into account influences of culture and ethnicity. Counselors may question clients about any inconsistencies in these top five factors, such as wanting a high prestige, high paying job but only wanting to complete high school to get it. Sometimes a resolution to the inconsistencies is not apparent until after clients have explored some of the alternatives available to them.

Stage 4, Generating Alternatives, and Stage 5, Obtaining Occupational Information

The next two stages of the career counseling process call for the client to generate some career choices (alternatives) based on preferences determined by the client during the previous stage and to conduct research on those career choices. Clients will need to do their own research, with motivation from the counselor. Motivating clients to do the work of gathering information may involve including family and friends in the process. The client may have friends and family with computer access the client may not have. The client's parents or spouse may be interested in some of the careers the client needs to research and may be happy to help with the research. In this way, the search for information becomes a group project and clients—especially those from collectivist cultures—may be more inclined to participate in data collection. Some clients will abhor library research, so the counselor will need to find alternative approaches to information gathering that will meet that client's learning styles:

Luis is motivated to research the two areas he is interested in, but to sustain his motivation, Ivy encourages him to get Harry, Luis's Anglo partner of five years, involved. Harry is an attorney and is well established in his current firm. He is concerned about the possibility of moving on Luis's behalf because he feels very accepted as a professional gay man by his own co-workers. Therefore, Harry is most interested in knowing where the jobs are located for the careers Luis is considering. He is also concerned about the annual salaries of Luis's potential jobs, and about the time it will take for Luis to be trained. Luis is interested in learning more about Latinos in these fields—how they got started, how successful they are, and so forth. Luis and Harry meet with Ivy to share the information they have gathered.

Stage 6, Making Choices

The time comes in most career counseling situations when the client must make a career decision. Decision-making styles are typically individual, but to help clients discover their own decision-making styles, most counselors try to teach their clients decision-making skills. Sue and Sue (2003) have stated that because counselors operate from a linear model, their approaches to problem solving may be in conflict with those of people from other cultures. Some cultures entail problem-solving styles that are more holistic and harmonious than linear, such as Native American cultures. In fact, Sue and Sue state, "When American Indians undergo therapy, the analytic approach may violate their basic philosophy of life" (p. 112).

For many, career decision making is a cut-and-dried task, because they have eliminated so many careers from their spectrum of possibility that discussion of career choice is moot. Some have eliminated certain careers as applicable to them primarily because they do not have and do not see a way to achieve the skills necessary to enter those careers. Others may believe that there is so much discrimination in a particular field they wouldn't have a chance of prospering there (Herring, 1990; Arbona, 1990). Herr, Cramer, and Niles (2004) suggest that it is the career counselor's job to assure culturally different clients that they do indeed have choices and that they can overcome discrimination. The best strategy is to try to connect clients with role models from their own cultural groups who have succeeded despite the barriers:

Ivy and Luis do not discuss career decision making until his work with her has resulted in some resolution about how he will handle his family and cultural situation. Luis's decision-making style is rather impulsive. He has given Ivy several examples of how his decision-making style has been somewhat successful, but most of the time, he has ended up regretting his decisions. Ivy points out that the decision he made to come out to his family is anything but impulsive. Luis, therefore, can and has employed different styles to greater success than his impulsive preference for decision making would indicate.

Luis has enjoyed collaborating on his decisions and wants to include his partner, Harry, in the career decision-making process, since Harry will be the person most affected by his career choice. Harry is invited to the sessions involving the gathering and evaluating of career information and provides feedback on his perceptions of Luis's abilities, values, and desires. Both he and Luis agree that the ultimate decision is Luis's but that it is important that they both be able to live with it.

Stage 7, Making Plans

One of the final steps in the career counseling process is the job search, which is undertaken with the assumption that the client already possesses the skills necessary to actually perform the duties of the desired position. For ethnic minority clients, the job search can be very stressful. Unfortunately, one of the by-products of affirmative action is that there is a pervasive assumption among both employers and prospective ethnic minority employees that ethnic minority applicants are *not* qualified for certain jobs. This bias handicaps the chances of ethnic minorities getting hired, and if hired, it may prevent them from getting promoted. Even though illegal in most cases, other kinds of prejudice and discrimination may be encountered by members of all oppressed groups and may result in rejection after rejection or lead to the client accepting a lower position for less money. As a result, career counselors need to be available to help culturally different clients tap into their support systems and utilize coping strategies.

For some ethnic minority clients, coping may involve a discussion of spirituality or other indigenous healing strategies. Support systems may include family and friends, as well as spiritual role models. The career counselor should let clients discuss their religious beliefs and how these beliefs have helped them cope in the past. A counselor's knowledge and understanding of the client's religion will help make these discussions much more fruitful. For example, if a Muslim client reveals that the difficulties he experiences at his job revolve around demands that keep him too busy to say his midday prayers, and he has found his supervisor to be neither sympathetic nor accommodating, knowing that Muslims must pray five times a day will make this discussion more meaningful for both the client and the counselor.

Even though affirmative action has increased the number of ethnic minority groups in fields in which they were long excluded, affirmative action policies do not guarantee an individual a job. Affirmative action simply means, in many cases, that ethnic minorities have been included in the pool of applicants and perhaps interviewees. Employers simply have to make a case for why they have not hired the ethnic minority candidate or candidates. Clients need to understand that while they may get interviews, they must do well, including being prepared to successfully respond to any questions they may be asked. Clients should also be briefed on the types of questions that are illegal for prospective employers to ask (such as marital status, parental status, racial/ethnic background, place of birth). The reason these kinds of questions are illegal is to prevent prospective employers from using information against clients in hiring.

The counselor and client should work out a strategy the client is comfortable with if a prospective employer does happen to ask an illegal question, and the client should rehearse the response so that the client can recite it without anger or emotional upset. Clients should be encouraged to do research on potential employers regarding their hiring and retention of ethnic and cultural minority employees. Unfortunately, there are as yet no federal restrictions preventing discrimination against people because of their sexual orientation, so counselors should discuss this distressing matter and how to navigate its implications with their gay, lesbian, bisexual, or transgendered clients.

Luis is not yet ready to do a job search, but part of the planning stage was for him to determine how to approach his family about his sexuality. After much deliberation, he decides to come out to two of his cousins and his siblings. He will not swear them to secrecy but will tell them that he wants to wait a while before discussing his sexuality with the older members of his family. He believes that he is prepared to accept whatever reactions his family members may have because it will be such a relief to stop deceiving them.

Stage 8, Implementing Plans

When a client obtains a job, the career counseling process is not quite complete. Often a career change not only entails growth opportunities for clients, but also means clients will need to adjust to a new role within the family and community. Counselors need to help clients prepare for these new roles. This is especially important in cases of career changes among dual-career couples and clients with children, because the roles of all family members will be affected by career changes. Balancing career, family, and community are important for the well-being of all individuals, so an important part of the career counselor's job is to help clients realize appropriate balances between these life elements. This task becomes easier when the counselor has already integrated the client's family and culture into the career decision-making process. In addition to discussing the balance between career, family, and community, counselors should also discuss with clients how leisure time fits into the balance. Leisure activities are influenced more by socioeconomic status and perhaps ability status than by race, ethnicity, or sexual orientation. The more money clients have, the more opportunities there are for a greater variety of leisure activities. Whatever the income level, however, it is important that clients consider leisure activities as part of the lifestyle planning process:

Luis has decided that he will go back to school full-time, which has implications for Harry's lifestyle as well as Luis's. There will be a reduction in income, an increase in expenses (tuition, books, supplies), and a change in household responsibilities.

In their last session Luis reports that he has applied to a culinary arts school that has hours that will allow him to still work part-time in his current job. His employer is willing to be flexible with his schedule while he is in school. Luis and Harry have decided to allow Harry's younger sister to exchange housekeeping and cooking duties for a room in their house while she attends her first year at the university. They are both happy with the solution and feel confident that it will work out well.

GROUP CAREER COUNSELING

Before concluding this chapter, a few words need to be said about group career counseling, because the career counseling competencies include both individual and group career counseling. Group counseling is a more typical format for career education and decision making in school settings than in out-of-school settings. However, career groups are also effective for stress management, role exhaustion, and interpersonal problems that manifest themselves in the workplace. There are several reasons for the popularity of group counseling in career development:

- It works. Group career counseling can be as effective as individual counseling if test interpretation and feedback are given individually (Brown & Krane, 2000).
- The developmental nature of career counseling means that more people need it. In other words, psychotherapy is needed by only a few people, but all people go through the same developmental stages (e.g.., deciding on a career) so more people need career counseling than psychotherapy.
- It is efficient. More people can be served in a group than via individual counseling, and group counseling maximizes the counselor's time.
- It is the preferred intervention for some cultures. In fact, the groups that would benefit most from a group career counseling format tend to be collectivist in nature (e.g. Latinos/as and Native American) or those individuals who feel particularly isolated (gays, lesbians, and bisexuals, people with disabilities) (Gladding, 2003).

The group career counseling structure is somewhat different from that of individual career counseling. Because of the structured and pre-planned nature of career groups, group counseling does not entail all of the typical stages of the group counseling process. However, career groups may experience two or more of these stages.

The first stage, known as the forming or pre-group stage, is the domain of the career counselor. Counselors need to be certain that multicultural groups include more than one member of any oppressed group or that there is equal representation of a number of culturally different groups (in cases of culturally diverse groups), or that the group is homogeneous or made up of members of one specific group (in cases of groups consisting of one culturally different group, such as Latinas and Latinos, people with disabilities, gays and lesbians, and so forth). One of the main purposes of a group is that the clients within the group feel as if they have something in common with one another and that they will be able to connect. If one member of the group feels different from the others at the outset, then joining the group may be problematic to that person. On the other hand, if a group is homogeneous, there may be a sense of rapport, trust, and cohesion, but some of the benefits of a group can be lost if the members are too similar. Therefore, the general consensus of group experts is that the group be heterogeneous to maximize not only the diversity of ideas, but also to promote cultural understanding among group members (DeLucia-Waac & Donigian, 2004). It may also be useful for counselors to assess client collectivist values. Those who have the collectivist orientation would do well in a group. Otherwise individual career counseling may be more appropriate.

Once group members have been identified, group leaders typically provide a group orientation to help clients understand the group format, as recommended by many group work specialists (Bowman & DeLucia, 1993; Cummins, 1996). While the orientation session can be elaborate and include activities that introduce members to group strategies, counselors may alternately choose simply to explain the purpose, stages, and role expectations involved in group counseling. Importantly, the rules and guidelines for handling conflicts in the group need to be established. Also, it is important in the orientation or in the first actual group session to mention the multicultural make-up of the group, just as culture should be called attention to in individual counseling (DeLucia-Waac, 1996) and to model for the group appropriate behaviors for discussing differences.

Since most career groups are structured, formats for career groups have been created. Pyle's (2000) model includes four stages.

Opening Stage

In this first stage, clients get to know each other and the counselor, the rules of the group counseling process are established, and the counselor uses rapport-building skills to encourage clients to connect with one another and to create a safe environment. In a multicultural group, a challenge during this phase would be helping clients to get in touch with their similarities and differences while developing group cohesiveness. Rules will be very important during this phase, because although the group would want to talk about differences, members of the group would need to be protected from hurtful stereotypes and prejudices. In this phase, the counselor needs to get this message across to clients while simultaneously avoiding crippling client self-expression by making clients fearful of alienating one another. Counselors must make sure they monitor the group and encourage expression of real feeling of concern and confusion yet model how to ask questions and give feedback.

Investigating Stage

In this stage, clients discover many of their own characteristics through test-taking, clients learn about careers and the barriers they may find to some careers, and the counselor encourages, supports, and self-discloses. In a multicultural group, the challenge for counselors at this phase will be interpreting each member's test results differently, based on the available comparison groups. Also, if a client is not represented in the normative group for a particular test, then the counselor will need to decide whether or not to assign the test to the client and will need to figure out how to interpret the test results if the test is administered. The recommendation is that tests be interpreted individually, even if everything else is done as a group. This may be the best bet in a culturally diverse group.

Working Stage

In this stage, clients take in all the data presented to them and try to make sense of it, and counselors use skills such as accurate empathy, confrontation, and feedback. This is the stage when clients discover that they have either set their job prospect sights too high, or that they have a wealth of choices. Here is where group support becomes vital, and members of the group may be able to give one another a deeper understanding of their individual results. Clients are often excited about their career options. The challenge for counselors of multicultural groups at this phase is to be sure to give information for ethnic minority organizations for the professions the clients are considering.

Decision/Operational Stage

During this final group career counseling stage, clients support each other's plans, and counselors use termination skills, such as drawing conclusions and solidifying next steps. The challenge for counselors of multicultural groups at this stage is that decision making can be difficult in the context of a diverse group. Not only do cultures differ in terms of what they expect from their members, but individuals within cultural groups also interpret cultural teachings in their own ways. Participants can help each other out by asking hard questions about culturally specific rules. Responding to group members will help clients articulate their ideas and in the telling clarify matters in their own heads.

FINAL THOUGHTS ON SKILLS

Career counseling is a complicated process that, too often, has been misunderstood. As Crites (1981) pointed out, career counseling is more difficult than psychotherapy and is needed more than psychotherapy. It is more difficult because career counselors must not only master counseling skills to assist clients with personal issues but also must master skills specific to career development. Career counseling is needed more because everyone, especially members of oppressed groups, can benefit from assistance with career planning. The goals of this chapter are to assist readers in developing a greater understanding of the counseling process in general and, more specifically, to illustrate how to integrate the multicultural and career competencies in a counseling setting. Knowledge of cultural influences introduced in earlier chapters is essential for career counselors to integrate these competencies.

The career counseling process described in this chapter followed eight of the stages outlined by Yost and Corbishly (1987). Although the eight stages are the same for every client, multiculturally competent career counselors tailor their approach to complement each client's racial/cultural background and the client's individual perceptions of that background. Counselors must establish a caring and trusting relationship during the first stage of career counseling, by attending to the cultural traditions and expectations of their clients. Doing so reduces client mistrust of the counselor and allows for a smooth transition to the other seven stages of the process. A trusting relationship allows counselors to engage clients in the counseling process in every stage by openly addressing cultural and sociopolitical factors that either enhance or limit the client's career development.

The culturally competent career counselor is an entirely different practitioner from those in the past who used three sessions and left a cloud of dust. Today's career counselor needs an ability to think critically and to understand the complexity of the clients he or she sees every day. It is a difficult task, but once it is learned, integrating multicultural and career counseling skills can be useful with all clients.

REVIEW/REFLECTION QUESTIONS

1. One of the career counseling competencies addressed in the chapter is the ability to "identify and understand social contextual conditions affecting clients' careers." Identify at least five of those conditions that affect Luis's career. Discuss the contextual factors that you would personally find the most challenging if Luis were your client.

2. List some of the reasons why career and personal counseling should not be approached separately. Then, discuss how personal and career issues have been intertwined in your own life—paying close attention to those times when the demands of family, culture, and career were in conflict.

3. List the eight stages of career counseling covered in this chapter and the cultural issues that should be addressed at each stage.

[Handwritten margin notes:]
One in the same lifestyle affects career choice & vice versa
• leave rocks for education/career
• Med School - No b/c I want to have a family

REFERENCES

Abernethy, A. D. (1995). Managing racial anger: A critical skill in cultural competence. *Journal of Multicultural Counseling and Development, 23,* 96–102.

ACRN America's Career Resource Network (author) (nd). *National Career Development Guidelines,* acrnetwork.org/ncdg/documents/NCDG.pdf Retrieved August 25, 2006.

Allison, K. W., Echemendia, R. J., Crawford, I., & Robinson, W. L. (1996). Predicting cultural competence: Implications for practice and training. *Professional Psychology, Research and Practice, 27,* 386–393.

American School Counselor Association. (2002). *The ASCA National Model: A framework for school counseling programs.* Herndon, VA: ASCA Publications.

Arbona, C. (1990). Career counseling research and Hispanics: A review of the literature. *Counseling Psychologist, 18,* 300–323.

Arredondo, P., Toporek, R., Brown, S. P., Jones, J., Locke, D. C., Sanchez, J., & Stadler, H. (1996). Operationalization of the multicultural counseling competencies. *Journal of Multicultural Counseling and Development, 24,* 42–78.

Bingham, R. P., & Ward, C. M. (1994). Career counseling with ethnic minority women. In W. B. Walsh & S. H. Osipow (Eds.) Career counseling for women (pp. 165–195). Hillsdale, NJ: Lawrence Erlbaum Associates, Inc.

Blustein, D. L. (1987), Integrating career counseling and psychotherapy: A comprehensive treatment strategy. *Psychotherapy: Theory, Research, Practice, and Training, 24,* 794–799.

Bowman, V., & DeLucia, J. L. (1993). Preparation for group therapy: The effects of preparer and modality on group process and individual functioning. *Journal for Specialists in Group Work, 18,* 67–79.

Brammer, L. (1993). *The helping relationship: Process and skills* (5th ed.). Boston: Allyn & Bacon.

Brown, D., & Brooks, L. (1991). *Career counseling techniques.* Boston: Allyn & Bacon.

Brown, S. D., & Krane, N. E. R. (2000). Four (or five) sessions and a cloud of dust: Old assumptions and new observations about career counseling. In S. D. Brown & R. W. Lent (Eds.), *Handbook of counseling psychology* (pp 740–766). New York: Wiley.

Campbell, R. E., & Cellini, J. V. (1981). A diagnostic taxonomy of adult career problems. *Journal of Vocational Behavior, 70,* 645–647.

Constantine, M. (1998). Developing competence in multicultural assessment: Implications for counseling psychology training and practice. *The Counseling Psychologist, 26,* 922–929.

Corey, G. (2005). *Theory and practice of counseling and psychotherapy* (7th ed.). Pacific Grove, CA: Thompson Learning.

Crites, J. O. (1981). *Career counseling: Models, methods and materials.* New York: McGraw-Hill.

DeLucia-Waak, J. L., & Donigian, J. (2004). *The practice of multicultural group work: Visions and perspectives from the field.* Pacific Grove, CA: Brooks/Cole-Thomson Learning.

Evans, K. M. (1997). Wellness and coping activities of African American counselors. *Journal of Black Psychology, 23*(1), 24–35.

Evans, K. M., & Larrabee, M. J. (2002). Teaching the multicultural counseling competencies and revised career counseling competencies simultaneously. *Journal of Multicultural Counseling and Development, 30*(1), 21–39.

Evans, K. M., Rotter, J. C., & Gold, J. M. (2002). Synthesizing family, career, and culture: A model for counseling in the twenty-first century. Alexandria, VA: American Counseling Association.

Fernandez, M. S. (1988). Issues in counseling South Asian students. *Journal of Multicultural Counseling and Development, 16,* 157–166.

Flores, L. Y., & Heppner, M. J. (2002). Multicultural career counseling: Ten essentials for training. *Journal of Career Development, 28,* 181–202.

Flores, L. Y., Spanierman, L. B., & Obasi, E. M. (2003). Ethical and professional issues in career assessment with diverse racial and ethnic groups. *Journal of Career Assessment, 11,* 76–95.

Fouad, N. A. (1994). Career assessment with Latinos/Hispanics. *Journal of Career Assessment, 2,* 226–239.

Galassi, J. P., Crace, R. K., & Martin, G. A. (1992). Client preferences and anticipations in career counseling: A preliminary investigation. *Journal of Counseling Psychology, 39,* 46–55.

Gladding, S. T. (2003). *Group Work: A counseling specialty* (3rd ed.). Upper Saddle River, NJ: Prentice-Hall.

Gold, J. M., Rotter, J. C., & Evans, K. M. (2002). Out of the box: A model for counseling in the twenty-first century. In K. M. Evans, J. C. Rotter, & J. M. Gold (Eds.), *Synthesizing family, career, and culture: A model for counseling in the twenty-first century* (pp. 19–33*).* Alexandria, VA: American Counseling Association.

Hawks, B. K., & Muha, D. (1991). Facilitating the career development of minorities: Doing it differently this time. *Career Development Quarterly, 39,* 251–260.

Helms, J. E., & Cook, D. A. (1999). *Using race and culture in counseling and psychotherapy: Theory and process.* Boston: Allyn & Bacon.

Helms, J. E., & Piper, R. E. (1994). Implications of racial identity theory for vocational psychology. *Journal of Vocational Behavior, 44,* 124–138.

Herr, E. L. (1989). Career development and mental health. *Journal of Career Development, 16,* 5–18.

Herr, E. L., Cramer, S. H., & Niles, S. G. (2004). *Career guidance and counseling through the lifespan: Systematic approaches.* Boston: Pearson Education.

Herring, R. D. (1990). Attacking career myths among Native Americans: Implications for counseling. *The School Counselor, 38,* 13–18.

Highlen, P. S., & Sudarsky-Gleiser, C. (1994). Co-essence model of vocational assessment for racial/ethnic minorities (CEMVA-REM): An existential model. *Journal of Career Assessment, 2,* 304–329.

Ibrahim, F. A., & Owen, S. V. (1994). Factor analytic structure of the Scale to Assess World View. *Current Psychology: Developmental, Learning, Personality, Social, 13,* 201–209.

Ivy, A. E., D'Andrea, M., Ivy, M. B., & Simek-Morgan, L. (2002). *Theories of counseling and psychotherapy: A multicultural perspective* (5th ed.). Boston: Allyn & Bacon.

Jackson, L. C. (1995). Ethnocultural resistance to multicultural training: Students and faculty. *Cultural Diversity and Ethnic Minority Psychology, 5,* 27–36.

Krumboltz, J. D., & Coon, D. W. (1995). Current professional issues in vocational psychology. In W. B. Walsh & S. H. Osipow (Eds.), *Handbook of vocational psychology* (2nd ed.) (pp. 391–420). Hillsdale, NJ: Erlbaum

Lee, C. C. (1984). Predicting the career choice attitudes of rural Black, White, and Native American high school students. *Vocational Guidance Quarterly, 32,* 177–184.

Lowman, R. L. (1993). The inter-domain model of career assessment and counseling. *Journal of Counseling and Development, 71,* 549–554.

McFadden, B. (2003). Using bibliotherapy in transcultural counseling. In D. Harper and J. McFadden (Eds.), *Culture and counseling: New approaches* (pp 285–295). Boston: Allyn & Bacon.

McFadden, J. (1996). A transcultural perspective: Reaction to C. H. Patterson's Multicultural Counseling: From diversity to universality. *Journal of Counseling and Development, 74,* 232–235.

McWhirter, E. H., Torres, D., & Rasheed, S. (1998). Assessing barriers to women's career adjustment. *Journal of Career Assessment, 6,* 449–479.

National Career Development Association. (1997). *Career counseling competencies. http://www. ncda.org/pdf/counselingcompetencies.pdf.* Retrieved August 23, 2006.

Niles, S. G., & Pate, P. H., Jr. (1989).Competency and training issues related to the integration of career counseling and mental health counseling. *Journal of Career Development, 16,* 63–71.

Niles, S. G., & Harris-Bowlsbey, J. (2005). *Career development interventions in the 21st Century* (2nd ed.). Upper Saddle River, NJ: Pearson Merrill Prentice Hall.

Patterson, C. H. (1996). Multicultural counseling: From diversity to universality. *Journal of Counseling & Development, 74,* 227–235.

Pedersen, P. (1996). The importance of both similarities and differences in multicultural counseling: Reaction to C. H. Patterson. *Journal of Counseling & Development, 74,* 236–237.

Pedersen, P. (1999). *Hidden messages in culture-centered counseling: A triad training model.* Thousand Oaks, CA: Sage Publications.

Perrone, K. M., Perrone, P. A., Chan, F., & Thomas, K. R. (2000). Assessing efficacy and importance of career counseling competencies. *Career Development Quarterly, 48,* 212–225.

Ponterotto, J. G., Alexander, C. M., & Grieger, I. (1995). A multicultural competency checklist for counseling programs. *Journal of Multicultural Counseling and Development, 23,* 11–20.

Ponterotto, J. G., Rivera, L., & Sueyoshi, L. A. (2000). The Career-in-Culture Interview: A semi-structured protocol for the cross-cultural intake interview. *Career Development Quarterly, Vol. 49,* 85–96.

Pope, M. (1995). Career interventions for gay and lesbian clients: A synopsis of practice knowledge and research needs. *Career Development Quarterly, 44,* 191–203.

Pyle, K. R. (2000). A group approach to career decision-making. In N. Peterson & R. C. Gonzalez (Eds.), *Career counseling models for diverse populations: Hands-on applications for practitioners* (pp. 121–136). Belmont, CA: Wadsworth/Thompson Learning.

Ridley, C. R. (1995). *Overcoming unintentional racism in counseling and therapy: A practitioner's guide to intentional intervention.* Thousand Oaks, CA: Sage.

Ridley, C. R., Li, L. C., & Hill, C. L. (1998). Multicultural assessment: Reexamination, reconceptualization, and practical application. *The Counseling Psychologist, 26* (6), 939–947.

Roysircar, G., Arredondo, P., Fuertes, J. N., Ponterotto, J. G., & Toporek, R. L. (2003). *Multicultural counseling competencies 2003: Association for multicultural counseling and development.* Alexandria, VA: Association for Multicultural Counseling and Development.

Spokane, A. R. (1991). *Career intervention.* Upper Saddle River, NJ: Prentice-Hall.

Sue, D. W., & Sue, D. (2003). *Counseling the culturally diverse: Theory and practice* (4th ed.). Hoboken, NJ: John Wiley & Sons, Inc.

Thomas, D. A. (1993). Racial dynamics in cross-race developmental relationships. *Administrative Science Quarterly, 38,* 169–194.

Thomas, D. A., & Aldefer, C. P. (1989). The influence of race on career dynamics: Theory and research on minority career experiences. In M. B. Arthur & T. Douglas (Eds.), *Handbook of career theory* (pp. 133–158). New York: Cambridge University Press.

Whaley, A. L. (2001). Cultural mistrust and mental health services for African Americans: A review and meta-analysis. *Counseling Psychologist, 29,* 513–521.

Whiston, S. C. (2000). Individual career counseling. In D. A. Luzzo (Ed.), *Career counseling of college students: An empirical guide to strategies that work* (pp. 137–156).

Yost, E. B., & Corbishley, M. A. (1987). *Career counseling: A psychological approach.* San Francisco: Jossey-Bass.

CHAPTER 8
Social Action

Tamiko is a young Japanese American career counselor who has recently married and is considering starting a family. One morning on the way to work from her racially mixed working-class neighborhood, she notices a huge cloud of smoke coming from three or four blocks away. Not having time to investigate, she goes to work, but when she returns home that evening, she discovers that the smoke had been coming from a fire that destroyed one of the few affordable child care agencies in her neighborhood. Several parents are interviewed about their reactions to the fire, and Tamiko is saddened by their plight until one parent announces that the agency will be rebuilding as soon as they can. Although she never would have dreamed she would do it, Tamiko is one of the first volunteers for the rebuilding project. Every weekend for three weeks, she helps with the rebuilding. When it is over, she feels very proud and fulfilled. However, something the news commentator had mentioned the day of the fire has worried her the whole time she has been participating in the project. In her city, the number of affordable day care facilities is far exceeded by the demand. Tamiko decides that she needs to do more. In most of the households in her neighborhood, both parents have to work, and more expensive day care may mean losing their homes. Tamiko does some research and locates several organizations devoted to obtaining legislative intervention regarding the day care issue for families in her state. After attending her first meeting, Tamiko is satisfied that she is doing what she can do to bring about a needed change in society.

Social action is an essential component of multicultural career counseling. In recent years, there has been a steady increase in the number of articles calling on counselors to become involved in attaining social justice. According to Medea Benjamin of Global Exchange, social justice exists in "a society where all hungry are fed, all sick are cared for, the environment is treasured, and we treat each other with love and compassion" (Kikuchi, 2005, paragraph 1). Counselors can be particularly instrumental in working toward accomplishing the goal of social justice by taking social action. To define the term, social action is a commitment "to become agents of systemic change, to channel energy and skill into helping clients from marginalized or powerless groups break down institutional and social barriers to optimal development" (Lee, 1998, p. 7). Multicultural awareness and knowledge among counselors cannot help but impact their sense of social responsibility, and this naturally leads to social action (Lee, 1998; Lewis & Arnold, 1998).

In career counseling, social action involves working toward the elimination of discrimination against all oppressed groups in the career arena, whether that work entails eliminating discrimination in career training, hiring, or promotion. To achieve this goal, socially active counselors are committed to:

- Taking action to equalize the inequities in education for poor and ethnic minorities, as well as people with disabilities
- Taking action to equalize the inequities in applicant selection for jobs
- Working to defeat efforts to shut down affirmative action
- Taking action to break the glass ceiling that women, men of color, and others experience in the workplace
- Speaking out and lobbying legislators to include gays, lesbians, bisexuals, and transgendered individuals under civil rights protection

Tamiko's involvement in day care initiatives is a response to a core issue in career counseling—the realities of the dual-worker household. Counselors today can no longer enjoy the luxury of sitting in an office focusing solely on the client sitting before them while outside of the office oppressive policies exist that deny large segments of the population (including that client) their dignity and rights. A civil rights slogan of the 1960s illustrates this point: "If you are not part of the solution, you are part of the problem." Counselors, therefore, need to become advocates for social justice, which, as defined by Bell (1997, p. 3) is "full and equal participation of all groups in a society that is mutually shaped to meet their needs." Social justice includes a vision of society in which the division of resources is equitable and all members are physically and psychologically safe and secure.

Interestingly, the father of career counseling, Frank Parsons, set the standard for career professionals taking social action right from the start (Davis, 1969). Working with immigrants to help them find jobs in a newly industrialized world, Parsons believed that the unequal distribution of wealth and power required him to be tireless in his efforts to empower the poor and working classes. He helped establish the Vocation Bureau of Boston, which among its many goals worked to keep children from dropping out of school (Hartung & Blustein, 2002). Hartung and Blustein believe that counselor involvement in social action would bring career counseling back to the roots of its founder, Frank Parsons (Hartung & Blustein, 2002).

In addition to challenging the oppressive systems that exist outside of the counseling office, as many others since Parsons' time have advocated, Lewis and Arnold (1998) insist that counselors review the oppressive nature of the counseling profession itself and become activists for change within the profession. Although there has long been a call for social action among career counselors, there has at the same time been little change in the way career counseling is practiced. Fox (2003) and Vera and Speight (2003) criticize the profession for not taking the next step from awareness to action. Hurtung and Blustein (2002) agree, and further point out that even the theories of career counseling do not reflect a social justice agenda. For example, Liu and Ali (2005) have suggested that career counseling is biased when it focuses on college and professional careers for everyone. Li and Ali say that counselors therefore do not demonstrate an understanding of clients who do not possess this kind of ambition and thereby allow their own biases and classism to interfere with the counseling of the client. Fox takes this point further and points out that, worse yet, career counseling as a field is so focused on counseling individuals, on objective value-free science, and on the cultivation of moderate stances for tenure and promotion that it is unlikely much will change in the field.

SOCIAL ACTION COMPETENCIES

The good news is that both the multicultural and career counseling competencies address advocacy and social action, and various authors in the field have expanded upon this position. For instance, in her discussion of using multicultural counseling competencies as tools to address oppression and racism, Arredondo (1999) refers to the specific competencies that can help counselors reduce oppressive behaviors. She also points out several multicultural competencies that are particularly relevant to social activism:

- Culturally skilled counselors are aware of institutional barriers that prevent minorities from using mental health services (Sue et al., 1992, p. 482).
- Culturally skilled counselors have knowledge of the potential bias in assessment instruments and use of procedures, and interpret findings in a way that recognizes the cultural and linguistic characteristics of the clients (Arredondo et al., 1996, p. 69).
- Culturally skilled counselors should attend to as well as work to eliminate, biases, prejudices, and discriminatory context in conducting evaluations and providing interventions and should develop sensitivity to issues of oppression, sexism, heterosexism, elitism, and racism (Sue et al., 1992, p. 483).

Some of the NCDA competencies focus on social action, in a career development context:

- "Help the general public and legislators to understand the importance of career counseling, career development, and life-planning" (p. 6).
- "Impact public policy as it relates to career development and workforce planning" (p. 6).

- "Assist other staff members, professionals, and community members in understanding the unique needs/characteristics of diverse populations with regard to career exploration, employment expectations, and economic/social issues" (p. 6).
- "Design and deliver career development programs and materials to hard-to-reach populations" (p. 6).
- "Challenge and encourage clients to take action to prepare for and initiate role transitions" (p. 4).
- "Mount a marketing and public relations campaign in behalf of career development activities and services" (p. 5).
- "Advocate for the career development and employment of diverse populations" (p. 6).

To supplement these competencies in a manner more overtly focused on social justice, several advocacy competencies have been developed by ACA's Division of Social Justice to concentrate on specific skills that are needed to be effective as agents of social justice. Some examples of the counselor advocacy competencies include the following:

- Help the individual identify the external barriers that affect his or her development.
- Negotiate relevant services and education systems on behalf of clients and students.
- Develop an initial plan of action for confronting these barriers.
- Analyze the sources of political power and social influence within the system.
- Seek out and join with potential allies.
- Support existing alliances for change.

For the entire list of advocacy competencies compiled by the Counselors for Social Justice see: *http://www.counselorsforsocialjustice.org/advocacycompetencies.html.*

COMMITTING TO SOCIAL ACTION AND SOCIAL JUSTICE

Social action is thought by many to be the natural next step in multicultural competence. As one author put it, the counselor committed to social justice "seeks to transform the world, not just understand the world" (Vera & Speight, 2003, p. 261). Fox (2003), however, is pessimistic about the career counseling field's ever fully embracing social action and taking on a more radical stance, because career counseling students are not often encouraged to become socially active during their training programs.

Fox (2003) further suggests that resistance to social advocacy and social action occurs at times because it is a difficult task to change the deep-seated mindsets that come with any profession. Some professionals prefer to separate their politics from their work, while some are not sure how to combine work and politics. Additionally, one important theme that recurs throughout the literature on social action is that social action often involves risks that many are unwilling to take or that may be too costly for the counselor. If counselors decide to take stands on issues or if counselors become actively involved in protesting or supporting unpopular causes, they risk ridicule and harassment from others, both in the workplace and in the community (Lee, 1998).

They may also gain reputations as troublemakers and may alienate people who may be able to assist them. Blustein and colleagues (2005) also mention that true involvement in social justice may interfere with earning a livable income. Still, while Grieger and Ponterotto (1998) acknowledge that social advocacy may come with risks, they believe it is a necessary task. According to Gainor (2005), "understanding resistance to change is, ironically, necessary for change to proceed" (p. 185).

Though Blustein and colleagues (2005) suggest that career professionals have a moral imperative to become active in social justice because they are a privileged, educated group, Gainor (2005) argues that such an "awesome responsibility" may seem unattainable (p. 182). She suggests that even when privileged individuals want to change their passive behaviors to actively oppose oppression, they often resist doing so, not only because changing the system is a monumental task, but also because changing the system might mean losing privileged positions.

Even so, Gainor (2005) believes that losing privilege is a risk well worth taking, and using Evans's (1996) framework for implementing change, Gainor outlines the steps for career professionals to follow in the process of becoming activists:

- *Step 1.* Counselors must develop a strong enough sense of moral outrage that the outrage will overcome the fear of trying to change conditions faced by oppressed clients. The idea at work here is that counselors will be so upset about the state of affairs in society that to do nothing is a far more frightening prospect than to do something. Gainor suggests that the values outlined by Blustein and colleagues (2005) that come into play during this step are: (a) self-determination, or the power to foster in oneself and others the ability to attain mutually acceptable goals; (b) caring and compassion, not just for clients but for marginalized people who may not present themselves for mental health services; (c) collaboration and democratic participation, or the equitable opportunity for citizens to have peaceful and respectful input into their own lives; (d) human diversity, or the respect for and recognition and appreciation of diverse social identities; and (e) distributive justice, or the fair distribution of goods and opportunities among all social groups (Blustein et al., 2005, p. 150–151).
- *Step 2.* In this step, counselors move from a sense of loss to a sense of commitment. Gainor suggests that career agencies can facilitate this step by allowing counselors to embark on the change in their own time and in their own way rather than by mandate. She suggests that perhaps frank discussion of possible loss of privilege involved may facilitate acceptance and movement toward social action.
- *Step 3.* Counselors then gain competence in their new social action skills. Gainor suggests that this process should begin in preservice-level training. Students should be taught social advocacy skills in their career development courses as well as in specific courses on social justice.
- *Steps 4 and 5.* The last two of Gainor's steps toward becoming socially active are less focused on how to assist individual counselors, but rather focused on how the counseling profession can change. Step 4 is to "address the uncertainty and confusion that arises during the early stages of institutional reform," and Step 5 is to engage a critical mass of supporters to "exert pressure and appropriately use power [to] . . . assist in implementing a social justice agenda" (p. 184).

SOCIAL ACTION TRAINING

Once counselors are committed to actively pursuing social justice in their work with oppressed clients, and once the agency is also committed, social action training should naturally follow.

There is little evidence that social advocacy training is widely practiced. Although most professional counseling organizations advise counselors to become advocates, Blustein and colleagues (2005) point out that, although social justice has been discussed in the counseling literature by many, the majority of textbooks students learn from still focus heavily on one-on-one career services, not social advocacy. In fact, Fox (2003) argues that because the counseling field is so tied to existing institutions (schools, government agencies, hospitals), there is little chance that widespread social justice training will occur in the foreseeable future. Others are doubtful because counseling has traditionally focused on the specific issues of the individual while leaving community interventions to social workers and other professionals (Albee, 2000; Vera & Speight, 2003).

Goodman and colleagues (2004), however, have designed a training program to integrate social justice into training professionals. The program strives to assist "students to (a) gain an awareness of systemic factors impacting mental health, psychological growth, and career development, (b) experience collaboration across the professions, (c) do collaborative work, advocacy or indirect service with underserved populations, and (d) engage in the design, delivery and /or evaluation of preventive interventions" (p. 808). In designing the program, Goodman and colleagues required first-year doctoral students to spend six hours per week working in both urban and rural communities as well as courts, detention centers, community organizations and agencies, and public health departments to gain exposure to diverse groups. Through such exposure, students developed "skills in prevention, interprofessional collaboration, and advocacy" (p. 808).

Before beginning this program, Goodman and colleagues reviewed multicultural and family literature for evidence of discussion of social justice and found that it was indeed discussed and that the following themes were most integral to bringing about social justice: "(a) ongoing self-examination, (b) sharing the power, (c) giving voice, (d) facilitating consensus, (e) building on strengths, (f) leaving the client with tools" (p. 793). The program was therefore designed to provide students with opportunities to develop these skills.

According to Buckley (1998), there are three qualities of social justice: (1) the affective dimension, or the awareness of and sensitivity to the suffering that occurs under oppression, (2) the intellectual dimension, or the understanding of the causes and effects of oppression, and (3) the pragmatic dimension, or the practice of bringing about social justice. Counselor training texts typically address the first two dimensions, the affective and intellectual, while overlooking the pragmatic dimension. The activities that the students participated in and immersed themselves in during the project of Goodman and colleagues did address the pragmatic dimension. The students gained so much insight from the project that Goodman and colleagues (2004) recommend that more programs get their students involved in social action and integrate it into existing courses.

Keep in mind, however, that while learning projects such as the project of Goodman and colleagues are an excellent means for bringing social awareness into the forefront, and while social awareness can be helpful in treating the symptoms of social problems, awareness is not the same thing as social action. Serving soup to the homeless may go a long way in helping students gain a greater understanding of the plight of the homeless, but such an activity does not change the fact that there are homeless people in the first place. Social action is about doing something to change the institutions that through their policies cause these problems. For example, to reduce homelessness, students can learn to challenge the policies for early release of patients from mental hospitals, and they can help the homeless to secure jobs by educating employers.

Collison and colleagues (1998) have also outlined steps to train counselors in social action. They suggest first determining whether or not students want to engage in social activism and then, if so, determining each individual's style. They suggest the following pivotal steps in learning social advocacy:

(a) reading advocacy materials and other materials about social and organizational change
(b) understanding the law
(c) keeping track of changes that affect oppressed persons
(d) becoming a part of an existing advocacy group, either a larger, long-standing group such as the NAACP or the Southern Poverty Law Center, or a more locally-based organization devoted to promoting the welfare of the poor, the homeless, ethnic minority groups, gay, lesbian, bisexual and trangendered people, and/or people with disabilities

SOCIAL ACTION SKILLS CATEGORIES FOR CAREER COUNSELORS

Social action has been recommended by many as a practice in which all counseling professionals should engage. For career counselors in particular, there are specific social action skills that are of importance. Lee and Walz (1998) identified eight categories of social action skills for career counselors:

1. "Commit to acquiring greater competence in use of new information technologies as a means to further professional renewal" (p. 308)
2. Acquire and use "multiple assessment procedures that are designed to reflect adequately the characteristics of persons from an increasingly diverse and pluralistic society" (p. 309)
3. "Assign a higher priority in counselor education programs to the preparation of counselors as agents of social change" (p. 309)
4. Utilize outcome research "to promote greater public support of counseling and counselors" (p. 310)
5. Intervene into "[client] environments . . . to promote change . . . and . . . enhance the resilience and invulnerability of persons to [negative environments]" (p. 310)
6. "Help create alternatives and opportunities for people"

7. "Work to improve policies with respect to human welfare and development" (p. 311)
8. "Advocate at all levels of government" (p. 311)

Each of these categories will be addressed separately in this concluding section of the chapter.

Commit to Promoting Greater Access and Competence in the Use of Information Technologies

Casey (1998) explains that use of technology is something that most workers take for granted. However, a technology gap divides the social classes. Upper- and middle-class people have more access to technology and more control over the technology they use, while those in the lower classes tend not to have as much access to technology, and when they do have access, they are often held hostage by the technology. Casey provides an example of an upper-class white male who uses technology to make his work life more convenient, while a working-class mother is tied to her computer and headset to do her work. Moreover, lack of convenient access to technology in the home and at school affects the education of the woman's children and limits her family's access to career information. While it is true that today's public schools typically provide computer access to students, such access is limited, based on availability and demand. To help counselors get involved in reducing the "technogap," Casey recommended several programs that can help, including Computers and You, a program out of San Francisco that provides computer training to low-income and homeless adults and children, and Street-Level Youth Media in Chicago, which equips young people from low-income areas with the latest in communication technology (the Internet, teleconferencing, video technology). Casey and Sampson (1998) further suggest that counselors need to actively pursue funding for providing and improving technology for those caught in the technogap.

Sampson (1998) also challenges counselors to identify websites that are specific to the client's career development needs and to create self-help programs that can be used to track career development milestones. In all, the call is for counselors to push for more up-to-date technology in underserved schools, more computer training for underserved clients, and access to computers in more locations (such as in housing development offices).

Acquire and Use Multiple Assessment Procedures

Social action regarding assessment in career counseling may soon include advocating for the right of counselors who are not trained as psychologists to continue to use psychological tests with clients. There have been movements in several states to limit some or all testing—even those tests used almost exclusively by career counselors such as the Strong Interest Inventory—to doctoral-level licensed psychologists. Such a ban on master's-level counselors would have a major impact on career counseling and would reduce access to career services to members of many disenfranchised groups. Individuals unable to afford to see a psychologist for testing would have limited access to career guidance. A more far-reaching possible consequence of the above limitation would be that if diverse populations had limited access to standardized testing, there would be little incentive for test makers to change the standardization process to be more inclusive of diverse examinees. Counselors are therefore encouraged to become involved in the effort to find a workable agreement regarding the use of standardized tests by both counselors and psychologists, and to become involved in efforts to bring about reasonable legislation on this matter.

Assign a Higher Priority for Social Advocacy in Counselor Education Programs

The fact that so few students have received training in social action is unfortunate, but it is a reflection of how recently the desire for this competency has developed. The good news is that the Council for the Accreditation of Counseling and Related Educational Programs (CACREP), the Council On Rehabilitation Education (CORE), and the American Psychological Association (APA) now require advocacy training for new students, so a foundation for social advocacy skills among counselors has been set.

Until such standards are more pervasive in educational institutions as well as in the above-mentioned organizations, counselor educators can push to include social action as a part of the required career counseling course. Social action is particularly relevant to career development, because many of the oppressive conditions endured by clients are determined by their careers. Individual instructors should act as role models for social action by becoming knowledgeable about social action strategies and policies that impede social justice. They can start by taking a public stance on issues important to career counseling, such as affirmative action, bias in job placement and college placement testing, or bilingual education (Vera & Speight, 2003).

Intervene into Client Environments to Promote Positive Changes in Those Environments

Most of the strategies suggested by authors of social action literature fall under this category. Although the list of activities and behaviors that entail intervention is very long, only those most relevant to career counseling and development are discussed here.

Grieger and Ponterroto (1998) have provided a number of suggestions for advocacy intervention including:

- Defend causes for social justice in schools and in the workplace
- Confront co-workers who engage in discriminatory and harassing behaviors—especially at the time such behaviors occur
- Advocate for a zero-tolerance policy against discriminatory and harassing behaviors in the workplace
- When necessary, engage in formal protests against discriminatory policies

Other actions counselors might consider include soliciting the assistance of appropriate community organizations to oppose injustices, and becoming involved with community groups and individuals who are "fighting for change on their own behalf" (Lewis & Arnold, 1998, p. 59). Several authors suggest that counselors join forces with outside professional organizations to assist in facilitating social change (Brabeck et al., 1997; Hartung & Blustein, 2002). Career counselors, therefore, would not only be joining forces with other helping professionals, but also getting businesses, industries, and professional organizations run by ethnic minority and other disenfranchised groups involved in social advocacy.

To ensure that interventions further a social advocacy agenda, Prilleltensky and Prilleltensky (2003) suggest that counselors ask themselves (and others) the following questions:

- "Do interventions educate participants on the timing, components, targets, and dynamics of best strategic actions to overcome oppression?" (p. 200) In other words, do clients and others know the who, when, what, and how of the plan?
- "Do the interventions empower participants to take action to address political inequities and social injustice within their relationships, settings, communities, states, and at the international level?"
- "Do interventions promote solidarity and strategic alliances and coalitions with groups facing similar issues?"
- "Do interventions account for the subjectivity and psychological limitations of the agents of change?" (p. 200). The intervention should be appropriate for those advocating the change.

Help Empower Clients to Advocate for Themselves

Career counselors may begin the process of empowering clients to act on their own behalf by helping them recognize that the career challenges they experience often have a social cause. Empowering clients to act on their own behalf is a basic social advocacy skill counselors need to develop. Clients should be encouraged to initiate grievance processes when they experience discrimination on the job, and counselors should support them through this process. Also, counselors should supply clients with the information regarding resources and policies they need to take on such challenges. Support not only includes providing information, but also providing emotional assistance when clients become frustrated with the systems they are fighting. In addition, clients could be encouraged to get involved with (or establish if none is available) diversity-positive groups at their jobs, in their schools, or in their neighborhoods (Brabeck et al., 1997; Geiger & Ponterro, 1998; Hanson, 2003; Hartung & Blustein, 2002; Herr & Niles, 1998; Gainor, 2005). Consider, for example, the following scenario, which illustrates the importance of client empowerment:

Margarita, a career counseling intern, has a white female client, Susan, who is enrolled in the civil engineering program. Susan sadly informs Margarita that she is going to drop out of the program because she can't stand the negative attitudes of the students and faculty. Both students and professors either ignore or ridicule her ideas, fellow students leave her out of study groups, professors typically do not call on her in class, and she hates the way the teaching assistant looks at her every time she has a question during her laboratory classes. She says that it really is not worth the hassle, and there are other areas of engineering she can pursue without having to put up with this "old boy" stuff.

When Margarita suggests to Susan that she is being sexually harassed, Susan insists that no one has made a pass at her or anything remotely like that. Margarita explains that the hostile environment she is experiencing is, in fact, sexual harassment. Susan then gets really angry. Margarita and Susan discuss harassment further and Susan decides that she wants to do something about it. They work out a process for Susan to collect data by recording the time, place, and specifics about each incident over the next couple of weeks. She will then file a complaint. Although Susan had thought she would not change her mind about getting out of civil engineering, she now thinks pursuing both her degree and a sexual harassment claim will be positive moves not just for her, but also for the next woman who wants to enter the civil engineering program.

Work to Improve Policies with Respect to Human Welfare and Development

Regarding the skill of improving policies, it is probably most expedient for career counselors to begin by exploring detrimental policies in their own places of work before going on to explore the detrimental policies in place at other organizations. The types of actions counselors should take regarding improving policies include the following:

- Getting involved at the policy-making level, such as being on a committee that makes policy decisions on hiring, retaining, and promotion of employees. In such a role, counselors can also help resist the pressure from privileged groups to retreat from multiculturalism, and
- Getting involved in the evaluation of the organization's performance with diverse groups, and being involved with developing an improvement plan if needed (Greiger & Ponterroto, 1998).

Counselors who do not want to take on the entire organization may be willing to ensure that their own departments or programs are culturally diverse and sensitive (Greiger & Ponterroto, 1998). When working to improve policies outside of their own organizations, counselors may want to start by examining a local policy that affects their clients. For example, advocating for updating technology in an inner-city or rural school so that children can have better access to career information, or doing as Tamiko did in this chapter's opening scenario and finding an issue that is important in career development even if one does not have a client with such an issue at that time, are ways to improve policies.

Advocate at All Levels of Government

According to Herr (2003), career counseling has been closely aligned with governmental policy making throughout its history, and as such, career counseling has effected a great many governmental changes that have had positive effects on the career development of individuals from diverse backgrounds. Recent governmental-level policy changes that have been put into place largely through the efforts of career counselors include but are not limited to the School to Work Opportunities Act, the North American Free Trade Act, and the Workforce Investment Act. Herr notes that career counselors have failed to effectively convince governmental agencies to expand their notion of appropriate client base and types of problems for career counseling. Instead, only certain clients (such as unemployed, high school seniors or displaced workers) are being funded, and only certain career issues are addressed. However, because of their long-standing history of influencing governmental policies, Herr challenges career professionals to "take the lead for advocating for career counseling issues to policy makers at all levels" and "where there are voids in legislative provisions that affect particular subpopulations, career counseling professionals should advocate for amended policies and legislation" (p. 15).

FINAL THOUGHTS

A career counselor may assist clients in choosing a career that is perfect in terms of their personality, interests, and abilities, and may prepare those clients to meet the cultural challenges such careers may present to them, but such a counselor has only completed half the task. The task is not complete until society is confronted with changing its oppressive policies so that someday any child can be told truthfully, "You can be anything you want to be when you grow up." Therefore, counselors are encouraged to develop competencies in social action, commit to becoming involved in social action and social justice, and promote training in social action for counseling students. To paraphrase Derald Sue's presidential address to the APA's Division of Counseling Psychology, "How can we possibly live our lives, day in and day out, with the knowledge of our complicity in the dehumanization of [disenfranchised persons]? And how can we possibly sit at home and do nothing about it?" (Sue, 2005, p. 112).

REVIEW/REFLECTION QUESTIONS

1. Refer to the list of competencies developed by the Counselors for Social Justice, and discuss how being a culturally competent career counselor (using all the knowledge and skills discuss in this text) will or will not prepare you for acting on social justice issues.
2. Think of an injustice that exists in your community (such as overcrowded urban schools, lack of day care, limitations on mass transit, a legislature that has no representation by females or men of color). Discuss how these injustices influence career development of workers and future workers. Choose one of these injustices, and discuss how you would go about getting involved in social action to change the status quo.
3. Several authors mention counselor resistance to social action. List some of the reasons that were stated that counselors might resist involvement in social action. Discuss your reactions to each of the items on the list in terms of your own participation in social action. If you find yourself feeling resistant, what might you do to reduce that resistance?

REFERENCES

Albee, G. W. (2000). The Bolder model's fatal flaw. *American Psychologist, 55,* 247–248.

Arredondo, P. (1999). Multicultural competencies as tools to address oppression and racism. *Journal of Counseling and Development, 77,* 102–108.

Arredondo, P., Toporek, R., Brown, S. P., Jones, J., Locke, D. C., Sanchez, J., & Stadler, H. (1996). Operationalization of the multicultural counseling competencies. *Journal of Multicultural Counseling and Development, 24,* 42–78.

Bell, L. A. (1997). Theoretical foundations for social justice. In M. Adams, L. A. Bell, & P. Griffin, *Teaching for diversity and socials justice: A sourcebook* (pp. 3–15). New York: Routledge.

Blustein, D. L., McWhirter, E. H., & Perry, J. C. (2005), An emancipatory communitarian approach to vocational development theory, research, and practice. *Counseling Psychologist, 33*(2), 141–179.

Brabeck, M., Walsh, M. E., Kenny, M., & Comilang, K. (1997). Interprofessional collaboration for children and families: Opportunities for counseling psychology in the 21st century. *Counseling Psychologist, 25,* 615–636.

Buckley, M. J. (1998). *The Catholic University as promise and project: Reflections in a Jesuit idiom.* Washington, DC: Georgetown University Press.

Casey, J. A. (1998). Technology: A force for social action. In C. C. Lee & G. R. Walz (Eds.), *Social action: A mandate for counselors* (pp. 199–212). Alexandria, VA: American Counseling Association.

Collison, B. B., Osborne, J. L., Gray, L. A., House, R. M., Firth, J., & Lou, M. (1998). Preparing counselors for social action. In C. C. Lee & G. R. Walz (Eds.), *Social action: A mandate for counselors* (pp. 263–277). Alexandria, VA: American Counseling Association.

Davis, H. V. (1969). *Frank Parsons: Prophet, innovator, counselor.* Carbondale, IL: Southern Illinois University Press.

Evans, R. (1996). *The human side of school change: Reform, resistance, and the real-life problems of innovation.* San Francisco: Jossey-Bass.

Fox, D. R. (2003). Awareness is good, but action is better. *Counseling Psychologist, 31*(3), 299–304.

Gainor, K. A. (2005). Social justice: The moral imperative of vocational psychology. *Counseling Psychologist, 33*(2), 180–188.

Goodman, L. A., Liang, B., Helms, J. E., Latta, R E., Sparks, E., & Weintraub, S. R. (2004). Training counseling psychologists as social justice agents: Feminist and multicultural principles in action. *Counseling Psychologist, 32*(6), 793–837.

Grieger, I., & Ponterotto, J. G. (1998). Challenging intolerance. In C. C. Lee & G. R. Walz (Eds.), *Social action: A mandate for counselors* (pp. 17–50). Alexandria, VA: American Counseling Association.

Hartung, P. J., & Blustein, D. L. (2002). Reason, intuition, and social justice: Elaborating on Parson's career decision-making model. *Journal of Counseling and Development, 80,* 41–47.

Helms, J. A. (2003). A pragmatic view of social justice. *Counseling Psychologist, 31*(3), 305–313.

Herr, E. L. (2003). The future of career counseling as an instrument of public policy. *Career Development Quarterly, 52,* 8–17.

Herr, E. L., & Niles, S. G. (1998). Career: Social action in behalf of purpose, productivity and hope. In C. C. Lee & G. R. Walz (Eds.), *Social action: A mandate for counselors* (pp. 117–136). Alexandria, VA: American Counseling Association.

Kikuchi, D. (2005). What is "social justice"? A collection of definitions. Retrieved August 22, 2006 from *http://www.reachandteach.com/*.

Lee, C. C. (1998). Counselors as agents of social change. In C. C. Lee & G. R. Walz (Eds.), *Social action: A mandate for counselors* (pp. 8–14). Alexandria, VA: American Counseling Association.

Lee, C. C., & Walz, G. R. (1998). A summing up and call to action. In C. C. Lee & G. R. Walz (Eds.), *Social action: A mandate for counselors* (pp. 307–312). Alexandria, VA: American Counseling Association.

Lewis, J. A., & Arnold M. S. (1998). From multicultural to social action. In C. C. Lee & G. R. Walz (Eds.), *Social action: A mandate for counselors* (pp. 52–65). Alexandria, VA: American Counseling Association.

Liu, W. M., & Ali, S. R. (2005). Addressing social class and classism in vocational theory and practice: Extending the emancipatory communitarian approach. *Counseling Psychologist, 33*(2), 189–196.

Nilsson J. E., & Schmidt, C. K. (2005). Social justice advocacy among graduate students in counseling: an initial exploration. *Journal of College Student Development, 46*(3), 267–279.

Prilleltensky, I., & Prilleltensky, O. (2003). Synergies for wellness and liberation in counseling psychology. *Counseling Psychologist, 31,* 273–281.

Sampson, Jr., J. P. (1998). The internet as a potential force for social change. In C. C. Lee & G. R. Walz (Eds.), *Social action: A mandate for counselors* (pp. 213–225). Alexandria, VA: American Counseling Association.

Sue, D. W. (2005). Racism and the conspiracy of silence: Presidential address. *Counseling Psychologist, 33,* 100–114.

Sue, D. W., Arredondo, P., & McDavis, R. J. (1992). Multicultural competencies and standards: A call to the profession. *Journal of Counseling and Development, 70,* 477–486.

Vera, E. M., & Speight, S. L. (2003). Multicultural competence, social justice, and counseling psychology: Expanding our roles. *Counseling Psychologist, 31*(3), 253–272.

Name Index

Subject Index

Credits, continued from copyright page

Holland's Hexagon, page 100 From J. L. Holland, *Making Vocational Choices: A Theory of Vocational Personalities and Work Environments, 2e.* Published by Allyn and Bacon, Boston, MA. Copyright © 1984 by Pearson Education. Reprinted by permission of the publisher.

Figure 6.2 From Ridley, Li, and Hill, 1998. "Multicultural Assessment: Reexamination, Reconceptualization, and Practical Application," *The Counseling Psychologist,* Vol. 26, No. 6, 939–947. Copyright © 1998 by Sage Publications, Inc. Reprinted by permission of Sage Publications, Inc.

Individual and Group Counseling Skills, pages 144–146: Reproduced with permission from NCDA.

NCDA competencies, pages 173–174 Reproduced with permission from NCDA.

Five Steps for Career Professionals, page 175 Adapted from Robert T. Carter, 2005, "Social Justice: The Moral Imperative of Vocational Psychology," *The Counseling Psychologist,* Vol. 33, No. 2, p. 184. Copyright © 2005 by Sage Publications, Inc. Reprinted by permission of Sage Publications, Inc.

Categories of Social Action Skills, pages 177–178 Reprinted from Lee, Courtland C. and Walz, Gary R. (1998). A Summing Up and Call to Action. In Lee, Courtland C. and Walz, Gary R. (Eds.), *Social Action: A Mandate for Counselors.* (pp. 308–311). Copyright © 1998 The American Counseling Association. Reprinted with permission. No further reproduction authorized without written permission from the American Counseling Association.